"BOOM" YOU'RE WELL

With Cetyl Myristoleate

A NEW, NATURAL, ANTI-AGING DISEASE FIGHTER THAT
CAN CURE ARTHRITIS, HEADACHES, BACKACHES
AND ALMOST EVERYTHING ELSE

DOUGLAS HUNT, M.D.

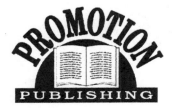

PROMOTION
PUBLISHING

"BOOM" YOU'RE WELL With Cetyl Myristoleate
By Douglas Hunt, M.D.
Copyright© 1996 by Douglas Hunt, M.D.
All rights reserved.

Published by:
Promotion Publishing
3368 Governor Drive, Suite 144
San Diego, CA 92122
1-800-231-1776

ISBN: 1-887314-28-8

Warning—Disclaimer
The author, publisher, endorsers, distributors, retailers, or anyone else associated with this book shall have neither liability, nor responsibility, to anyone with respect to any loss or damage caused, or alleged to be caused, directly or indirectly, by the information contained in this book. Please consult your physician before initiating the use of Cetyl Myristoleate as described by this book.

FOREWORD

An attractive, 36-year-old patient of mine with rheumatoid arthritis, feeling her life collapsing from a disease that deformed and tortured her, prayed for a miracle. . . she got it. . . and so can you. Does that sound too good to be true? Believe me, it's not! There is a certain magic in the story you are about to read and the information you are about to receive. The magic is **CETYL MYRISTOLEATE**—(say it: see-tul-meer-is-toll-ate). If you don't mind, I'm going to refer to it as **CMO** to make it easier on both of us.

We seldom hear the word "cure" around chronic diseases like arthritis. And that's because diseases like arthritis are so common that we almost come to think of them as normal.

Most people expect to get some kind of a chronic disease as they get older—it goes with the territory. And when it finally does arrive, we know we'll have to take our medicines and learn to live with it. And, although we don't dwell on it much, we more or less expect this problem to go on for the rest of our lives.

WELL, YOU CAN FORGET THAT OLD STEREOTYPE RIGHT NOW.

What if all the chronic diseases you've worried about, or suffered with, were actually eliminated. . . ALMOST OVERNIGHT?

What if the treatment was. . . ALL NATURAL?

What if there were few side effects. . . NO RISKS?

What if it were relatively speaking. . . INEXPENSIVE?

What if the results of the treatment lasted. . . THE REST OF YOUR LIFE?

WOULD YOU CALL THAT A MIRACLE?

If you have one of these diseases, or know someone who has. . . don't put this book down!!!

RHEUMATOID ARTHRITIS	OSTEOARTHRITIS
BURSITIS	TMJ
DIABETES	MS
LUPUS	ARTERIOSCLEROSIS
HYPERTENSION	CARDIOVASCULAR DISEASE
FIBROMYALGIA	PSORIASIS
LOW BACK PAINS	CROHN'S DISEASE
IRRITABLE BOWEL	ULCERATIVE COLITIS
ACHING FEET OR LEGS	MIGRAINES
EMPHYSEMA	FIBROCYSTIC DISEASE
TENSION HEADACHES	HEADACHES
ECZEMA	SCIATICA
FIBROCYSTIC BREASTS	DEPRESSION
SACRO-ILIAC PROBLEMS	CARPAL TUNNEL
BRONCHITIS	TENDONITIS
ATOPIC DERMATITIS	TENNIS ELBOW
PROSTATIS	LEPROSY
SCLERODERMA	ANY T-cell dependent, AUTOIMMUNE DISORDER

TABLE OF CONTENTS

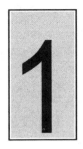

CAN CETYL MYRISTOLEATE
CURE EVERYTHING?

CETYL MYRISTOLEATE will probably be seen as **the** most important find of the twentieth century.

It was discovered over 25 years ago at, <u>of all places</u>, the National Institute for Health, but until 1995 virtually no one had ever heard of it. . . why? Why was it kept a secret? That's just one of the many mysteries in this amazing story revealed, for the first time, in this book.

IS _CMO_ A UNIVERSAL REMEDY?

This book is about _CETYL MYRISTOLEATE, what it is, how it works, and the numerous diseases that it cures or nearly cures_—the list is almost endless. _CETYL MYRISTOLEATE_ (say it: see-tul-meer-is-toll-ee-ate) is one of nature's fatty acids, <u>which I will refer to from now on as _CMO_</u>.*

---

* I was given permission to use the word _CMO_, trademark name, by KNOLLWOOD, Inc. The only manufacturer whose product I have used and feel confident with.

Is *CMO* a universal remedy?

Yes!

But let's be clear. I'm not suggesting that *CMO* is the cure for everybody and everything, though *CMO* will be tremendously beneficial to 90 percent of those with chronic diseases.

Many of you will go into prolonged remissions after using *CMO.*

When you introduce a new product like this, it must fit into some slot in the reader's library of ideas. *CMO* is so *unique* it's going to be tricky, but I'll make it as easy as I can.

CETYL MYRISTOLEATE, THREE KEY QUESTIONS

This entire book answers three key questions. Just what is *CETYL MYRISTOLEATE?* What is *CETYL MYRISTOLEATE similar to*? And what does *CETYL MYRISTOLEATE do*?

This chapter answers the first two questions.

I won't spend much time on *CMO*'s chemistry (what it is), because it won't mean much to you unless you're a chemist.

I can clarify things faster if I compare *CMO* to better known agents.

Comparisons to current therapeutic methods similar to *CMO* is the only way you'll ever understand how *CMO* works, so a review is important. We're going over this information lightly to start, and then coming back with more detail in Chapters 23 and 24, *AFTER* you have seen *CMO* in action.

These two areas aside, the rest of the book is essentially dedicated to what *CMO* does.

I interviewed over a hundred and twenty people as I wrote this book, not to mention the patients I personally treated. I'll tell you some of their stories as they told them to me.

Now let's take a brief look at what *CMO* is.

WHAT IS CETYL MYRISTOLEATE?

CETYL MYRISTOLEATE is a simple (natural) chemical that looks like this,

$$Cis\text{-}CH_3(CH_2)_{14}CH_2OOC(CH_2)_7CH=CH(CH_2)_3CH_3$$

It's an oil. In one form **CETYL MYRISTOLEATE** is thick like peanut butter, in another it looks like a waxy powder. You might shudder when I mention the words *oil* or *fat*. Well, don't. I promise you this is one of the good kinds. I'll rephrase that. *It's one of the GREAT KINDS.*

First of all, *CETYL MYRISTOLEATE* is a molecule made from two items: cetyl alcohol and myristoleic acid.

Cetyl alcohol was originally derived from sperm oil as a fatty alcohol: white in color and waxy in appearance. Now cetyl alcohol is made out of palmitic acid. Its main use, up until recently, was as an ingredient in cosmetics. It's been used in perfumes, face creams, lotions, and lipsticks.

It's also a *surface acting agent* and is found in detergents and pharmaceuticals. As a *surfactant* it retards evaporation of water and has been spread over reservoirs, and sprayed on plants.

Surfactant means *surface acting agent*. That means it reduces the viscosity of a fluid. Acting as a lubricant, it makes sticky, molasses-like fluids slick, so things can slide back and forth easily. Probably the most common statement made by those who take *CMO* is that they feel looser, less tight.

Myristoleic acid, the other half of the molecule, is found in sperm whales too, and in the oil glands of beavers, in vegetables and kombo nuts. It can be considered a marine oil like cetyl alcohol. It has been used in cosmetics, soaps and perfumes as well as being an additive in foods, just as cetyl alcohol.

CMO is a combination of cetyl alcohol and myristolic acid. Their individual *surface acting qualities* mesh to make a super *surfactant* we call **CETYL MYRISTOLEATE.** There is one question that must be addressed before we continue. How can one nutrient modify so many diseases?

IS THERE SUCH A THING AS A UNIVERSAL CURE?

The thought that one substance could cross all boundaries and influence virtually every chronic disease of any importance, smacks of chicanery. And yet, the idea that a single system could be behind all causes and all cures of disease is *not a new idea at all.*

From time to time, scientists have offered theories that unify the disease process. T.N. Lee, for example, set forth such a theory in Medical Hypotheses (May 1994). In his article, "Thalamic Neuron Theory: Theoretical Basis for the Role Played by the Central Nervous System in the Causes and Cures of All Diseases", Lee argues that since the central nervous system is involved in sending and receiving messages for most, if not all, of the body's activities, then it must be the supreme control center for all of the body's homeostatic functions. Therefore the central nervous system *has to be* involved in the causes and cures of all disease.

Lee starts his paper with the observation that present day therapies for the most important diseases of our time are largely palliative rather than curative. I would agree with that, wouldn't you? He goes on to say that this is because the disease process itself is poorly understood. Obviously, if it were better understood then we should have less disease.

It's important you recognize the possibility that one substance **_can have_** enormous effects on multiple diseases.

For uninformed readers, the concept of one-cure-fits-all seems bizarre. The concept seems especially strange to people, knowing as they do, that medicine has divided itself into so many specialties: cardiology, rheumatology, pulmonology, etc.

Is it any wonder that the understanding of what chronic disease is, really gets blurry with this division of medical effort?

CHRONIC DISEASES, MORE ALIKE THAN YOU THINK

Chronic disease is much simpler than it is made out to be, as you will see. That is to say, an inflammation in the kidneys is not dissimilar to an inflammation of the joints. A dysfunctional immune system that attacks the nervous system of those with multiple sclerosis can be identically dysfunctional when it attacks another group of tissues that make up, say. . . the joints.

Medical specialists want to cluster themselves around some particular anatomical site. They are more secure being one-organ-doctors. The point I am making is that it is a mistake to believe diseases are all different because they have different names.

WHY MY JOINTS, NOT MY SKIN?

The next logical question is: why does a disease process, such as inflammation, choose to attack one organ or system at a time?

The answer is equally logical: it depends on an individual's genetics and environment.

Genetically speaking, each person is born with strong and weak organs and strong and weak systems. A virus or a toxin will find the going easy in the genetically vulnerable liver of one individual or the weakened kidneys of another.

Take psychological stress, for example. Why does mental stress cause one person to react with depression, another to be angry, aggressive and destructive, another to be frightened and cowering, and another to be obsessive compulsive? Why do troubled people all choose different defense mechanisms to protect themselves?

The answer is, because everyone responds differently to stress, depending on their genetic strengths and weaknesses, and depending on the type of stress in progress.

The various anatomical systems will respond in the same way, and with the same diversity of symptoms. Doesn't that seem logical?

Let's say you have a headache and your neighbor tells you he has bursitis. On the surface you're talking about two different diseases, but in reality both of you may be talking about the same disease process. The inflammation is simply presenting itself in two different locations in the body. The common denominator is the inflammation—it's just not in the same system.

2

HOW DOES CMO WORK?

The quickest way to familiarize yourself with an unknown product is to compare it to something you do know about. The closest I can come is to pick two products which match the effects of *CMO,* but on a lesser scale. My two selections are: the essential fatty acids, fish oil and flax seed oil, and oral vaccines that relate to the autoimmune system. Most of the readers will have some knowledge of essential fatty acids, while everyone has had some experience with a vaccine. Nearly everyone in this country knows that the way you vaccinate is to inject the killed organism that you want your body to develop antibodies against.

Since the injected organism is dead you won't get polio, for example, but your body will think it has to defend itself against polio, so it will make enough antibodies to defend itself. When the real organism shows up the body is ready for it.

In autoimmune disease the body is generally building antibodies against a protein that is a specialized part of yourself. It may be some tissue in joints or the myelin protein that surrounds nerves. In this case the body must interfere with the production of antibodies, not make them. You can see this is going to be tricky. I'll tell you all about it as we go.

THE FIRST SIMILARITY; *CMO* AND THE ESSENTIAL OILS

When I first heard about *CMO* I was skeptical, to say the least, but since it was a natural substance I left the door open for a change of mind. Reports of its successes were unbelievable.

I decided to investigate and, soon after, because of what I had learned, I decided to write a book.

When you write a book like this, you need to know all there is to know about your subject. The problem here is there is virtually nothing in the literature that even remotely relates to this marvelous substance.

When I started my search I couldn't find any research directly involving *CMO* so I broadened the search. As I probed around for some common thread, one name kept popping up—fish oil. Yes!! Fish oil for diabetes, fish oil for hypertension, fish oil for arthritis, fish oil for congestive heart failure, and on and on.

As well as being a food, fish oil is one of nature's medicines. It is an unsaturated essential fatty acid. Specifically, there are three natural forms of essential fatty acids: flax seed oil, evening primrose oil and fish oil (which is usually salmon or a mixture of marine oils).

During my research, I made a very exciting find. Essential fatty acids are helpful for every one of the diseases that I knew were benefited by *CMO*. I learned that *successful clinical trials* had been conducted using the oils, in disease after disease.

It is true, then, that nature does have a remedy for virtually all types of diseases. *CMO* is connected to as many chronic diseases as fish oil. And **CMO** will do everything that fish oil can do... only better.

If **CMO** is an oil, as I believe, or very close to one, then it is the *Godzilla of oils*. Whatever the other oils (flax, EPO, and fish oil) can improve, **CMO** can improve a thousand times over.

If fish oil can improve irritable bowel syndrome by 10% or 20% as it has been shown to do, then **CMO** can improve it 50% to 70%. If fish oil can improve foot pains by 10% as scientific studies have already proven, then **CMO** can improve it 80% to 100%. If fish oil can improve arthritis by 10% to 30%, then **CMO** can cure it, as I have seen it do.

THE ESSENTIAL OILS AND MULTIPLE DISEASES

Here's what Gray and Martinovic have to say about essential fatty acids in their paper published in Medical Hypotheses (August 1993), entitled, "Essential Fatty Acids and Chronic Fatigue Syndrome."

Abnormal fatty acid balances, they say, *are found in every chronic disease*.

The authors hypothesize that changes in the ratios of the essential fatty acids are the normal responses to stress, but if the stresses are prolonged or excessive, then essential fatty acid systems may become permanently and unpredictably hypo-responsive owing to factors such as receptor down-regulation and developing deficiencies.

After some unknown period of time, many of the homeostatic systems become deranged and held in that state by minor stressors. For example, in chronic fatigue syndrome there is a hyper- and hypo-responsiveness in immune function as well as dysfunctions in the involuntary nervous system. It has been found that adding essential fatty acids and maintaining the intake can reverse the hyper- and hypo-responsiveness.

Changes in essential fatty acid metabolites have been studied in many diseases: lupus, chronic granulomatous leukemia, allergies, arthero-genesis, thrombosis, arteriosclerosis, peripheral vascular disease, gout, psoriasis, atopic dermatitis, coeliac disease, chronic inflammatory bowel disease, cystic fibrosis, rheumatoid arthritis, adult respiratory distress syndrome, obstructive pulmonary disease, tuberculosis, multiple sclerosis, fibrositis of all types, and the list goes on.

The essential fatty acids are constantly in short supply. The reason is that the body's chronic need for more EFAs is caused by an inextinguishable inflammation which burns on and on, day after day, week after week, year after year. This sort of endless stimulation leads to depletion of the essential fatty acids.

The enzyme, delta-6-desaturase, which is responsible for metabolizing the essential fatty acids, has been postulated to be deficient in chronic fatigue conditions. Delta-6-desaturase is quickly depleted by a number of physical insults such as:

1. Excessive mono-unsaturated fats in the diet (nuts);
2. Excessive saturated fats;
3. Too much sugar in the diet;
4. Excessive alcohol intake;
5. A high cholesterol diet;
6. Starvation and malnutrition;
7. Zinc and magnesium deficiencies;
8. Severe viral infections;
9. Mononucleosis, Epstein-Barr;
10. Diabetes;
11. Radiation;
12. Not taking care of oneself as one ages and;
13. Stress.

Once this chronic imbalance in fatty acids starts, a series of small stresses is all that is needed to keep it going.
The right nutrient can improve chronic diseases, because all chronic diseases have the same imbalances.

CMO is *SIMILAR TO* the essential oils in that when it is used for treatment, it reduces inflammation and pain and extends range of limb motion. But there is one big dissimilarity. The essential oils must be taken for years or a lifetime, while **CMO** need only be taken for a few weeks. Sometimes one or two capsules may be necessary afterwards as a booster.

THE SECOND SIMILARITY

CMO's modifying actions are similar to the EFAs, but it's not *exactly* like them. I was struggling for an explanation for some of these discrepancies when I stumbled upon the answer. **CMO** is like an *oral tolerizer too!*

Chapter 23 will provide extensive background on oral tolerization. I'll just give you a simple explanation here.

An oral tolerizer is a highly refined food extract, made from a specific animal part. This extract is fed to an individual with an autoimmune disease, such as multiple sclerosis. The immune system is stunned and the disease process slowly stops.

The different between oral tolerization and **CMO** is that in the former, one has to manufacture a specific desensitizing substance for each disease. For example, if you wanted to desensitize an individual to the antibodies that cause MS you would use MBP, myelin basic protein, which is refined from beef. The material is given orally, and must be continued on an indefinite schedule.

The problem with oral tolerization is, you have to make up a different protein for each disease, and that is precisely why this excellent treatment is still unavailable through normal channels. Scientists are still arguing over manufacturing techniques, and other details related to the treatment process.

In case you are wondering "When did this all happen?" let me tell you. Research has been ongoing with oral tolerization since the 1960s. And even though research has been highly productive it has never been passed on to the clinicians for the reasons I've just mentioned (see Chapter 10 for an exception to this statement). If that frustrates you, join the crowd. Researchers debate and recalculate while people suffer and die. It certainly does point out each person's priorities.

CMO seems to have many of the characteristics of both an oral tolerizer and an essential oil, that is, it acts somewhat like an oil, and yet it may stun the immune system so rapidly that it could almost be an oral tolerizer. Amazingly, it affects every disease equally well. With *CMO*, there is no need to manufacture special materials for each distinct disease. *CMO* is ready to work right out of the bottle.

One has to believe *CMO* may be a universal immune modulator of monstrous proportions under these circumstances. Perhaps it's one of nature's best-kept secrets.

At the same time *CMO* does all these wonderful things, there are no side effects to speak of.

IMMUNE SYSTEM DYSFUNCTIONS AND INFLAMMATION

The body's immune system defends the body from attack in many ways. One way is to make antibodies that attack and destroy invaders. But what if it gets confused? What if the immune system begins to see a part of the body as the enemy? What if it attacks? Tissues are now being damaged and destroyed, and we have an autoimmune disease on our hands.

As part of the strategy, white blood cells produce antibodies to attack a tissue, the cells create an inflammation. Unless something turns them off they never stop the attack. They are merciless and relentless, like terminators. What remains then is a static disease, a smoldering inflammation. This chronic inflammation then slowly devours the organ it is attacking.

The real culprits are a certain subset of white blood cells that make antibodies. They're called lymphocytes. Some are made in the bones and some in the thymus gland. They have different functions, depending on where they're made.

The T cells (from the thymus) and the B cells (bone lymphocytes) are the fire starters that perpetuate the inflammation. They provide the gasoline (the eicosanoid hormones) and the antibodies.

Humans use drugs to deal with this problem, of course—powerful, toxic ones.

But nature has already given us remedies too; unfortunately, we ignore that fact.

Excellent research has pointed out alternatives to drugs, but doctors resist the change.

The two alternatives I'm talking about are essential oils, such as fish oil, and the oral tolerization program. Hundreds of research projects have proven the effectiveness of the essential oils, and yet you never hear about them. And dozens of research papers have proven oral tolerization programs to be successful, but when did you last read about them?

Both of the above remedies reverse or eliminate many aspects of the autoimmune reaction (self-destruction). They both reverse inflammation (I'll give you the technical details on these two systems in Chapter 8).

TO SUMMARIZE. Keep in mind that **CMO** has the same effects as the essential oils, only stronger.

NATURE'S FIRST TEAM

In animals, essential oils of the n-3 series are nature's first team of firefighters. They dash to the scene and douse the fire. To some degree they also suppress the production of the fire starters (T and B cells).

Essential oils are great against small fires but only fair against big fires (chronic severe inflammations). That's because the essential oils are working from the ground up. They do most of their work *after* the fires have started. They can weakly hold off the fire starters (T and B cells), but they can't stop them. . . or the disease.

The oral tolerization approach attacks the problem from the top. It turns off the production of fire starters. Oral tolerization disables the machinery that makes specific antibodies and virtually negates, through some complex chemistry, the activity of the T and B cells toward specific tissues. In a sense it shuts down the factory that makes auto-antibodies.

CMO DOES BOTH JOBS

CMO can do what essential oils do, and many times over. It can also do what oral tolerization does. The disease being treated usually goes into permanent remission. If the reversal is not complete, at least it improves the condition of the disease by huge percentages.

There is an uncanny parallel between what the researchers have uncovered and what I, as a clinician, have observed. Although I have seen essential oils improve the symptoms of arthritis, I have never seen them reverse arthritis. On the other hand, I have seen *CMO* erase the symptoms of rheumatoid arthritis in as little as three weeks.

SURFACTANTS—HARDNESS/SOFTNESS

There is another effect of **CMO** that I want to emphasize. Its incredible power as a surfactant. Essential fatty acids have surfactant qualities, but nothing like **CMO**'s.

Throughout the book I will frequently refer to **CMO** and the essential oils as thinning oils. Fluidizing is only one of their qualities, but in my mind it is one of the most important ones.

It's true that too much thinning can be as bad as too much thickening, but the body always errors on the side of the latter. The body seems to harden as a natural course when left to itself. Thinning oils need to be taken daily to offset this hardening process.

The wrong foods, saturated fats, rancid oils, too much meat, high cholesterol foods, can accelerate the hardening process too.

Hardening is associated with disease and aging. Thinning is associated with health and youth. When I speak of thinning oils again you'll know I mean a quality of an oil that makes things healthier, smoother and more functional.

With aging, the body accumulates more of the hardening, cholesterol-type fats as part of the normal aging process. There is no doubt that the fatty acid balance is being lost.

It matters not whether it's the fluid in the blood or the fluid in the cell walls. Things slow down and hang up when the viscosity thickens to molasses, becoming ever more sticky, tacky and adherent.

The thinning effect, on the other hand, makes things more like liquid gel.

Obviously, a gel cannot hold a shape like lard can, and that's why the body needs a little of both. Your body is supposed to keep a balance between soft and hard, to find a middle ground. Disease and aging knock the balance off center toward hardness—this correlation between disease and aging is closer than most people recognize.

Let's look at an example of the surfactant effect in action.

CMO is a specific agent against rheumatoid arthritis, an autoimmune disease. And yet it also benefits osteoarthritis which is not an autoimmune disease. *CMO's* primary benefit to osteoarthritis, then, is probably as a surfactant. It helps the mild inflammation, but most of all it loosens and removes the stiffness of osteoarthritis almost overnight. The fact that it works so rapidly on stiffness makes a strong case for *CMO* being an incredibly strong surfactant.

3

THE SCOPE OF CMO

Let me give you a feel for the scope of this nutrient, and a sense of how many lives it will improve.

ARTHRITIS

It is 98% effective against both osteo- and rheumatoid arthritis. By "effective", I mean it will either cure the disease outright, or at least leave the recipient greatly improved.

There are over 50,000,000 Americans with osteoarthritis and another 6,000,000 with rheumatoid arthritis. Current treatments for these two diseases are highly toxic.

There are 6 billion people on earth, most of whom are going to get arthritis someday.

This same nutrient is 80%-100% effective against chronic low back pain or any back pain for that matter. Low back pain is the second leading cause for physician visits in this country. It is **the only reason** for the existence of chiropractic care. At first glance, that might not seem too important, but keep in mind chiropractics is the second largest medical profession in the world. The chiropractor's primary function is to service the 50,000,000 Americans who frequently complain of low back pains; billions of dollars are spent yearly on this ailment. Billions more are lost annually because of work absences. And low back problems are the number one cause for workers compensation claims.

The 15,000,000 people who suffer from chronic foot and ankle pains could experience almost total and rapid relief with *CMO*. The National Records on Health and Medicine show foot pains to be responsible for a high percentage of medical visits, and a frequent cause for employee absenteeism.

There seems to be a sundry of myopathies reported lately, fibromyalgia being the most common. Sometimes it's hard to tell where fibromyalgia stops and chronic fatigue syndrome starts. All I know is that they both fade under the healing balm of *CMO*.

Autoimmune diseases may partially respond to *CMO*. I will have more to say about it later in the book. *CMO* should be combined with antioxidants and other nutrients for the best effects against this class of disease. Currently 10,000,000 women and men are ill with autoimmune diseases.

TMJ and carpal tunnel syndrome often are alleviated, if not cured by *CMO*. I will present my own case histories as well as those of others.

When it comes to old sports injuries with their lingering pains—*CMO* shines. Commonly, there will be damage to the joint or tissue involved, and yet the pains may totally disappear after using *CMO*. When the coaches find out how great *CMO* is, they may give it to their athletes *to prevent injury*. Joint movements, after taking *CMO*, are so flowing and easy that performance may be enhanced. The likelihood of injury is also less.

Today 15,000,000 people have emphysema. Emphysema

and similar lung diseases improve dramatically with *CMO*. The scar tissue remains, but the inspired volume of air is increased by as much as 35%, and most importantly the progress of the disease is slowed or stopped.

Diabetics experience a reduction in insulin usage, especially if *CMO* is combined with other antidiabetic nutrients. In some cases insulin may be discontinued entirely. A pre-diabetic patient of mine, saw his blood sugar return to normal within one week after starting *CMO*.

This patient had a second problem. A year and a half before I saw him, he developed Bells palsy, and the left side of his face slumped. It was especially crucial for him to find a solution, because his position required him to give frequent television interviews. Needless to say, he was embarrassed. The palsy improved 25% during the first week of *CMO*, and another 25% in the next two weeks.

My diabetics have often reduced their insulin, and many have discontinued it altogether. There are 14,000,000 diabetics in this country who would just love to find a way to reduce or eliminate insulin.

CMO is being used by the elderly because it is an aphrodisiac, a euphoric, and an energizer (Not to mention an anti-arthritic). I am using *CMO* on many patients who say it helps their memory and increases their energy. Today, there are 31,000,000 people over 65, and 100,000 over age 100.

39,000,000 women in the United States have headaches, another leading cause for time off work. Headaches have been responding very well to *CMO,* especially if the headaches are migraine or the tension type.

Next, hypertension: so far *CMO* has improved the blood pressure of many who try it. If these early studies continue, we can add another 15,000,000 possible users to our list.

CMO works on other diseases too.

It's improving inflammatory bowel disease, Crohn's disease and colitis. About 11 million people have bowel problems.

Half the families in this country have pets. *CMO* is dynamite for pets. After all, they develop the same diseases that we do, including arthritis. I'm sure that every pet owner in the country will be thrilled to hear about *CMO*.

In a number of cases *CMO* has been helpful for psoriasis and eczema. It's a little too premature to say how many people will see improvements, but we know some will.

CMO IS JUST A NUTRIENT

CMO is a simple nutrient, not a drug. This makes its discovery even more exciting because, unlike drugs, *CMO* usually doesn't cause serious side effects.

CMO is an oil (fatty acid) much like fish oil, except that it's a hundred times more powerful. It may not work exactly like fish oil but its effects are identical and stronger.

The relationship is clear then: if extensive and academically acceptable research shows that an oil from fatty fish can alter a wide variety of seemingly dissimilar diseases, then so can a MEGA MEGA oil such as *CMO*.

CMO is a medium-chained fatty acid which closely resembles flax seed oil, evening primrose oil and fish oil. Oils in this class all have the same effects on tissues. Until *CMO* came along, fish oil was considered more effective than flax seed or evening primrose oil, which is why it was used more often in research.

Because *CMO* is a natural substance derived from food, with little potential for profit, scientific research has lagged.

Clinical interest, however, is now heating up, especially among alternative care physicians.

Throughout the book, I will quote the numerous studies which support this alternative care approach. I will also present over 50 case histories that demonstrate the colossal power of **CMO**.

I am aware of the controversy this book is bound to cause, but it will be a godsend for handicapped people and for many others who live with constant pain.

But, **CMO** is by no means an exclusive treatment for the seriously ill. It will relieve or eliminate most of the common aches and pains the rest of us feel.

And another thing—whatever **CMO** fixes—STAYS FIXED.

And it does its job with as few as 100 capsules of powder.

Many who've taken **CMO** have been free of rheumatoid arthritis for as long as nine years. And yet, of the several thousands who have used it, there have been no reports of side effects.

I have labeled **CMO** the "WD 40 of nature."

At this moment newsletters from alternative care physicians are telling readers about this substance. Word of mouth will soon send it onward and the net will begin to buzz. The excitement that this product is causing *cannot be contained.*

CMO is monumental in its benefits.

When you see a gnarled, ancient-looking man brought to you in a wheelchair walk through the door standing perfectly erect a month later, you know you've seen something akin to the transformations of Lourdes.

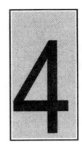

THE DISCOVERY

Before I tell you the story of **CETYL MYRISTOLEATE's** discovery, let me introduce you to its power.

Ken is a 72-year-old man who has been limited to his wheelchair until recently. That's because he used to have rheumatoid arthritis. A laboratory test that showed him to be actively rheumatoid, the sedimentary rate reverted to normal. You may call that "a remission" or whatever you like: the fact is he is not now suffering from any of the symptoms of rheumatoid arthritis. He still has many of the bony deformities to remind him of the past, but he doesn't have pain or swelling, and he can move his joints through most of their previous ranges. And he can walk!

Two years ago he was in constant pain, so much so he couldn't sleep more than 30 minutes during the night without waking up in pain. Naprosyn and the other NSAIDs were not working. Cortisone did work but he was afraid to take it on a continuous basis. The gold treatment had failed and he was scheduled to go on tomoxifen. Tomoxifen is excellent for rheumatoid arthritis, but it is also an extremely toxic drug that can cause tissue damage as well as cancer. Ken had good reasons to avoid it.

Ken was very depressed for two other reasons. He had the beginnings of diabetes and hypertension. At 71, his quality of life was about at an end. Those serious health problems seemed to point toward a painful, torturous, premature death.

When Ken heard about *CMO* he was skeptical but hopeful. He went for it with his last desperate prayer, especially since it didn't involve any risks.

He was better after three weeks. His joints were moving 50% farther, and they appeared less inflamed and swollen. His overall pain level had dropped 70%. He continued to improve over the next few weeks—less pain, more mobility—until he was substantially recovered.

Ken has been in remission now for over a year, but several times within the year, when the pains seemed like they might return, Ken took more *CMO*. He found that a single capsule of *CMO* was all that was necessary to eliminate any suspicious symptoms.

IT'S NOT JUST ARTHRITIS

This book is not about rheumatoid arthritis or any disease in particular. It's about chronic disease in general, the whole concept of how chronic diseases come about, and how to cure them. It's about the long-term diseases that have previously been considered incurable, especially the ones having to do with pain and inflammation.

CMO will be the focus of attention, of course. This newly-discovered nutritional supplement may improve the way medicine is practiced around the world.

CMO is a strange and relatively rare, but natural material. It's found in the oil glands of male beavers, in a complex mixture of waxes, called castor fiber. It is also found in sperm whale oil... AND IN SWISS ALBINO RATS... AND THAT'S WHERE THIS STORY BEGINS.

THE DISCOVERY

The first time doctors ever heard of *CETYL MYRISTOLEATE* was when the Journal of Pharmaceutical Sciences published an article in late 1993 entitled, "Cetyl Myristoleate isolated from Swiss albino mice: an apparent protective agent against adjuvant arthritis in rats." The article had been developed by the Department of Pharmacology, Medical College of Virginia.

There has been no follow-up research to date. Unfortunately, this article caused no great stir in the scientific community.

The story actually began 25 years earlier when Harry W. Diehl was an obscure researcher at the National Institute for Health. What he discovered in 1971 was never revealed until 25 years later when he presented it in the November 1993 Journal of Pharmaceutical Sciences.

Mr. Diehl was assigned the project of creating arthritis in a strain of rats in order to test a drug. Fortunately for us he used a strain of rats called, for the National Institute of Health's general purposes, Swiss Albino Rats.

When scientists investigate a disease like arthritis, they just can't set mouse traps around hoping to catch old, arthritic rats, they have to create arthritis in normal animals. They choose animals, usually rats, and inject them with a chemical which they know from experience creates the disease they need.

An injection of heat killed Mycobacterium Butyricum (also known as Freunds Adjuvant) will create arthritic symptoms (inflammation, pain and swelling) in susceptible mice. Diehl was apparently unaware the Swiss Albino rats were a strain that couldn't be made arthritic. When Diehl injected Mycobacterium Butyricum into the Swiss Albino rats they did not get arthritis.

Researcher Diehl's curiosity was raised: he needed to know why these rats resisted arthritis. But apparently there was no interest expressed by those above him, because they refused to fund further research.

Diehl's curiosity was greater than his obstacles. He decided to fund his own research as best he could.

Given the fact that there were limited finances, as well as limited time and space to do the work. it was fortunate for you and me that Mr. Diehl took up the challenge. His experiments were not as controlled as would have been desired, but they did clearly point out a direction of great promise.

Mr. Diehl's first project went like this:

Ten normal, general purpose, Swiss Albino mice were injected with 200 mcgs of mycobacterium butyricum (Freund's adjuvant). 10-20 days later there was no noticeable swelling in the legs or paws.

A second group of 5 mice were injected in the left hind paw. Again, after 10-20 days no discernible changes were seen.

Diehl then necropsied the rats and searched their chemicals for the one that protected them from arthritis.

Mr. Diehl worked hard for months, and eventually he did hit paydirt. He extracted hundreds of substances from the Swiss Albino rats, but only one, *CETYL MYRISTOLEATE,* worked.

The next fortunate finding was that producing *CETYL MYRISTOLEATE* was extremely simple. It was a combination of cetyl alcohol and Myristoleic acid, easy to reproduce in the laboratory.

Now he held this golden substance in his hands. A real triumph for a man working alone. And now it was time to find out what this puppy could do.

A different strain of mice was then used, one known to be susceptible to the effects of the toxin. 10 male mice of the Sprague-Dawley strain were injected with *CETYL MYRISTOLEATE* two days before they were given the toxin. A second group of nine rats received only the toxin. Both groups were observed for two months with respect to weight, hind and front leg swelling.

All rats receiving Freund's adjuvant (the toxin) alone developed severe swellings of the joints. 10-13 days after the toxin was injected, the rats in this group suffered the pains of full blown arthritis, but, in addition, their normal weight gains were poor. They gained only 14 gms during a 32-day period of observation. They were morbid and lethargic as well.

Those receiving Freund's adjuvant plus *CETYL MYRISTOLEATE* gained an average of 80 gms during the same period, and suffered no arthritic symptoms.

Diehl decided to synthesize his own *CETYL MYRISTOLEATE* instead of undertaking the laborious process of extracting *CETYL MYRISTOLEATE* from rats.

A second test was run using the synthetic *CETYL MYRISTOLEATE* which he had constructed in his laboratory.

Diehl used the same protocol of injections on a second group of mice, using the synthesized material.

The response was exactly the same as was seen with the original extract. The rats protected by *CETYL MYRISTOLEATE* were symptom-free, while all those in the control group developed arthritis and failed to thrive. It was a deeply satisfying moment for Diehl.

The livers were checked in several of the animals with arthritis and found to be swollen to 30% above normal.

Mr. Diehl concluded, at the end of his experiments, that **CETYL MYRISTOLEATE** alone gave nearly perfect protection against arthritis.

As Diehl speculated on the results, he came to the conclusion that the miraculous effects were a result of some powerful form of immune modulation. Today, that theory seems to predominate every time the subject of **CETYL MYRISTOLEATE** comes up.

I can see why he came to that conclusion and I agree it is one of the effects. Despite the lack of research so far, I'm sure **CETYL MYRISTOLEATE** has other, and possibly more powerful effects. I have expressed my views throughout the book.

Diehl has said that he informed his superiors on numerous occasions of his findings, but was rebuked each time without explanation. He says he has no idea why his findings were disregarded, but he suspects the impact of this agent might negatively affect some major financial interests. Whatever the reasons, there was no further research.

But the story is not over.

Diehl patented his ideas for the use of **CETYL MYRISTOLEATE**. Apparently he lacked the interest or business skills to exploit his discovery and so this valuable information was slipped onto a shelf and forgotten until Diehl himself began to develop arthritis. His doctor confirmed the diagnosis and wrote him a prescription for an anti-inflammatory drug. Diehl was told he would probably have to take the prescription for the rest of his life.

That did it! Diehl knew he didn't want to spend the rest of his life on drugs, and particularly the anti-inflammatory drugs that are known to become harmful eventually (I will review these toxic, long-term side effects in Chapter 25).

Diehl believed that the drug treatments were worse than the disease, so he decided to review his almost-forgotten files and use **CETYL MYRISTOLEATE** to treat himself. He made up a batch of this magic potion and gave himself an injection.

Diehl wasn't sure it would work but he knew it was harmless and he was hoping for some improvement. He was right on both counts—he didn't have side effects and the potion worked like a charm.

In a matter of weeks Diehl's arthritis disappeared so completely it was as though he had never had it. His doctor was shocked to find Diehl symptom-free on his next visit. Many years later Diehl's doctor sent a letter to the editors of the Journal of Pharmaceutical Science and confirmed that Diehl did indeed have moderately severe osteoarthritis, but it had disappeared by his second visit, and Diehl did not seem to be suffering any side effects. The doctor never saw arthritic signs in Diehl again.

Diehl's arthritis apparently stayed in permanent remission.

But there's more: the story does not end here.

There were added, positive side effects too. Diehl's long-term chronic headaches disappeared, never to return. His chronic bronchitis said "sayonara" also. For the first time in years he felt he could breath normally.

DIEHL'S SECOND PATIENT

Diehl's next patient was his daughter. He injected **CMO** hoping to relieve her chronic low back pains, firmly believing his product was perfectly safe. She had complete, apparently permanent, relief without side effects, just as he had.

Now the story gets a little fuzzy. Diehl retired from his research position, but was unsuccessful in exploiting his findings in business. He continued giving it to friends and neighbors when they complained of various ailments. Symptom relief occurred 98% of the time, according to Diehl. He has said over and over that the symptoms disappear and don't return.

Suffice it to say, over the years, 800 to 900 of Diehl's acquaintances were given the product and the results, according to Diehl, continued to amaze even him. People seemed to have few qualms about taking it since it was a natural product, and so they took it for a vast variety of complaints. Many of these complaints were far afield of arthritis but, in spite of that, the individual's condition usually responded to it.

Meanwhile, many of his earlier volunteers remained free of arthritis. At this writing, some have been arthritis-free for 9 years.

Probably the most difficult thing to believe about this substance is the tiny amounts needed to produce results. A hundred capsules of powder spread out over a few weeks is a small price to pay for a lifetime of relief.

All the pain, swelling, inflammation and restriction of motion. . . GONE. . . never to return. . . WOW!!

Harry Diehl's name should be placed in history books. Now over 85, Diehl is not in the best of health. It may be too late for him to be publicly acknowledged for his astonishing efforts, but let us hope that his name will eventually be recorded for what he's done.

CETYL MYRISTOLEATE was gradually discovered by alternative care practitioners, who, always on the lookout for good, natural approaches to healing, had heard about some of Diehl's successes. Alternative care physicians began to use *CETYL MYRISTOLEATE* on a variety of conditions and were just as astonished by the results as Diehl's friends had been.

CMO IS THERAPEUTIC

Let's take another look at *CMO*'s effectiveness.

BILL

Bill woke up one morning because he had to go to the bathroom, As he reached the halfway point his wife *screamed.* Bill was *walking*! This was his fourth day on *CMO*. For you and me, walking is the usual mode of travel to the bathroom, but not for Bill. He creaked to the bathroom with his cane because he had rheumatoid arthritis. He wasn't quite ready for a wheelchair yet, but he was getting there fast.

The other thing Bill's wife noticed was that she hadn't been kept awake all night by his constant tossing and turning. Bill couldn't sleep an hour without waking with a pain somewhere. Without pain, he slept through the night, which allowed his wife to do the same.

Bill is a graphic artist who depends on the computer for his livelihood. His hands were gradually freezing up. It wasn't just the lack of movement in the fingers, it was all that pain he suffered when he tried to use them. And then there were the other pains to distract him, the ones in the shoulders, his back, his knees, and the ones in his left hip and right foot. He couldn't even raise his arms above his shoulders because of the stiffness.

He remembers now, about all that stiffness and tightness. The same symptoms that others with rheumatoid arthritis complain about so often.

CMO saved Bill's graphics career. Until he used *CMO* he was becoming so disabled he was planning to apply for permanent disability. Bill is backed up with work now. He doesn't use a cane. He sleeps through the night, and he has no pain or restriction of motion.

Two other unexpected things happened. The severe

burning headaches that he used to experience have disappeared, and his hypertension is gone. Before he took **CMO,** his blood pressure, without medication, was over 200. Now his blood pressure reads somewhere near 130 over 75.

I've seen this sort of thing before—multiple symptoms disappearing all at once. But that stands to reason, doesn't it? When one's overall health is compromised by a disease, it is likely that other systems will become unbalanced, too. And if multiple systems can all be unbalanced at once, then they can all be rebalanced at the same time.

CMO'S BASIC EFFECTS

When you think of **CMO** you can think of three basic effects. First and foremost, *it removes inflammation*. Second, *it removes pain* and, third, *it makes physical movements easier* by lubricating the joints and moving surfaces.

Let me describe what I consider to be the typical response to **CMO** in a case of rheumatoid arthritis.

RUTH

Ruth is a 67-year-old lady who suffered the ravages of rheumatoid arthritis for 24 years. She dumped her arthritis in January 1996 after taking a two-week course of **CMO**. If you should happen to pass her on the street or have a casual conversation with her, you would never guess she used to be a cripple, shuffling around with a walker, looking like death warmed over.

Back in 1995 Ruth could barely sleep because of the constant pains. She tossed and turned all night and woke up exhausted. It took forever to get warmed up and loose enough to get out of bed. Her feet were swollen so badly she could rarely get her shoes on. All of the knuckles of her hands, her elbows, her knees, her shoulders and her back were painful, inflamed and swollen. She could not bend her fingers. She couldn't raise her arms above her chest.

Ruth's knuckles looked huge. There were "big balls" on her elbows, as she described them. Her knees were knobby, and her fingers and toes were twisted out of alignment. In a word, she was a mess. Poor Ruth was suffering with the multiple deformities so common to those who have severe rheumatoid arthritis.

There was one other thing about Ruth which is also common to those with this kind of arthritis. She could tell when the weather was going to change by the extra pains in her joints. She would have made a darn good weatherperson because she could tell you every time it was going to rain. . . without fail.

Over time, most of the drugs Ruth had taken lost their effects, but in early 1996 she was taking methotrexate, cortisone and relafen, an anti-inflammatory drug. These drugs were just barely holding the pain and inflammation at bay. She certainly wasn't comfortable or improving; in fact, she was getting worse.

Ruth also had constant wheezing and frequent asthma attacks for which she used the usual medications, plus oxygen. Her third problem was a stomach ulcer. Her ulcer was the result of years of using aspirin and anti-inflammatory drugs, which she said had chewed up her stomach pretty bad.

Ruth finished her treatment with *CMO* in the middle of January 1996, suffering no side effects from *CMO*.

Since the middle of January 1996, Ruth has been free of all of her signs and symptoms of rheumatoid arthritis. She has absolutely no joint pains or sore spots. She has full range of her limbs. All of her "knobs" have disappeared, including the big ones on her elbows, some large unusual ones under the skin near both wrists, and the two huge bunion-like knobs under the ball of her big toes. ***They are all gone!!***

Ruth's lungs have cleared of wheezing and she has not been experiencing asthma since January when she first took ***CMO***.

Another thing happened which came as a pleasant surprise. She does not have her ulcer any more! All of her abdominal pain is gone at last. Ruth is grateful beyond words about her recovery from arthritis, but she thinks the absence of her ulcer is the best of all, because that darn ulcer really made her life miserable.

One final note about Ruth. She has lost her weather vane. Her joints won't tell her when it's going to rain anymore. Well, I guess ***CMO*** can't do everything.

5

BACKING UP YOUR CMO

CMO is terrific! But, CMO is not perfect. Some individuals are cured for life after using it, while a few don't respond as well as expected. I noticed this as I studied CMO's effect on different people with the same disease. It looked to me like CMO could use a little help at times. I added other nutrients to CMO, and was pleased to see the new combinations producing more consistent responses, but CMO was always the center piece with its helpers at its side.

There is a clear precedent for this outcome. In studies where EFA's or coenzyme Q 10 were added to pain or anti-inflammatory medicines the supplements clearly potentiated the drugs. The improvements were so strong, in fact, the medicines could be reduced.

Nutrients notoriously support one another, so it should come as no surprise that CMO, as great as it is, can be strengthened with the addition of other natural items. Most nutrients require enhancing coenzymes for maximum effectiveness. I have listed supporting nutrients for CMO throughout the book.

Over the last 35 years I have used many so-called natural anti-inflammatories and have been disappointed with most of them. As you pass through each chapter in this book you will find the aids to *CMO* that have, in my experience, lived up to their reputation. So as not to confuse you, I have listed only one or two for each disease. I have often been confused when an author lists 40 antidotes for each ailment, as though the reader had any idea which would be best for you. I have simply picked the best that I know of even though it might not be every doctors choice.

I suggest you consider using the supporting nutrients at the same time you use *CMO* in order to maximize the potential for success. If you don't you may find yourself purchasing a second supply of *CMO*. There are other considerations too. Sometimes *CMO* needs to be used over a longer period of time. Let us hope you are among the majority of individuals who respond strongly to *CMO*.

Don't give up if you are in the minority. If you fail to try long enough or hard enough you may overlook an extremely powerful treatment. It's hard to find good answers to chronic health problems, don't pass over this great product too quickly if your response is a little slow, it's loaded with possibilities.

A WARNING ABOUT SPERMICETI!

THERE ARE COMPANIES THAT CLAIM TO HAVE THE ORIGINAL FORMULA FOR CETYL MYRISTOLEATE, BUT THEY DO NOT. ONE CLUE TO THE FAKES IS THE USE OF A CHEMICAL CALLED SPERMICETI. SPERMICETI IS AN EXTREMELY INFERIOR BASE CHEMICAL WITH WHICH TO MAKE CETYL MYRISTOLEATE. MYRISTOLEIC ACID IS THE HIGHEST QUALITY BASE, IS EXTREMELY DIFFICULT TO FIND AND IS VERY EXPENSIVE. BUT IT MUST BE USED AS THE FOUNDATION FOR CETYL MYRISTOLEATE, OR THE

PRODUCT WON'T WORK, AND I DO MEAN IT WON'T WORK, AND THERE GOES YOUR MONEY DOWN THE DRAIN.

THE ONLY COMPANY THAT I KNOW OF THAT USES MYRISTOLEIC ACID AS THE BASE FOR *CMO* IS "KNOLLWOOD, INC." 1-800-249-7816. I HAVE CONFERRED WITH THE QUALITY CONTROL OFFICER FOR THIS COMPANY AND AM CONFIDENT THE PRODUCT IS FULL STRENGTH.

The only other source for high quality **CETYL MYRISTOLEATE** is Mr. Diehl's family, and I have no address for them at this time.

I have no financial relationship with either source.

SHOULD YOU CONTINUE YOUR CURRENT MEDICATIONS AFTER USING *CMO*?

I have advised my patients to do so if they notice any returning symptoms, but *CMO* should also be restarted. Usually the returning symptom will disappear in a day or two, then you can discontinue both of them. The use of medications does not undermine *CMO* and visa verse.

CMO DOES NOT WORK ON ALL BACK PAINS, HERE ARE TWO EXCEPTIONS

One almost unknown, but fairly common cause of back pain is herpes genitalis. This virus migrates throughout the body and attaches itself anywhere it likes. When the virus is reactivated it creates an acute inflammation. It's favorite area is somewhere along the back.

This virus may also appear as a boil on the buttock, hips or thighs. It may even migrate into the brain and cause severe headaches.

If you've overlooked this possibility you might want to try a large dose of the amino acid lysine, just to see if your back pain is caused by herpes (lysine relieves herpes symptoms). If it is herpes the pain will leave within an hour.

A second common cause for a mystifying back pain is food allergies. *CMO* is not effective against food allergies.

The first patient that drew my attention to this was a middle-aged lady who was constantly searching for relief from an unrelenting back pain. For years, the pain defied everything she tried. I asked her if she was eating any particular food repeatedly. After a thoughtful moment she replied—oranges. I told her not to eat oranges or any citrus fruit for a week, then she was to eat 6 oranges in one day.

When she returned her back pain had disappeared, and so had her addiction to oranges. She said the pain faded slowly after stopping the oranges. But it came back like a sledge-hammer blow on the day she ate 6 oranges. The pain was so bad she had to go to bed.

CAN I CONTINUE *CMO* FOR AN INDEFINITE PERIOD IF I NEED TO?

My experience is that some individuals are going to need *CMO* for long periods, especially those who receive tremendous pain relief. I talked to the manager at Knollwood, Inc. And he agreed to make special arrangements for those of you who need ongoing supplies of *CMO*. The number to call is 1-800-249-7816.

WHERE MAY I FIND THE OTHER SUPPLEMENTS LISTED IN EACH CHAPTER?

Most of these items are in your local health food store. Alternative care products can sometimes be found in specialty pharmacies that cater to this market. The more "difficult-to-find" items are listed in the last chapter of this book.

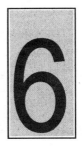

MENDING THE ARTHRITIC

What image do you get when you think of getting older? Most people see, in their mind's eye, an old man or woman bent over and feeble. It's the picture of a person shriveling up. . . shrinking. Look closer at the hands of this imaginary person. Do you see the gnarled joints and bony fingers? Do you see them shuffling along slowly. . . unsteadily? If you were asked for an opinion on the cause of that stooped appearance and the frozen joints would you answer. . . arthritis? I know you would.

You would link arthritis to the elderly like everyone else. . . and view it as inevitable.

Up to now you would have been right. . . but not anymore. There are big changes in the wind for millions of Americans.

Who are these Americans?

They are the 50+ millions of Americans with arthritis, most of them women. For women, arthritis is the number one cause of activity limitations over the age of 45. This information comes from the National Health Interview Survey.

Much time and energy has gone into studying the costs of

caring for people with chronic diseases like arthritis. The government needs to know what the cost will be to take care of these people. It's doubly important when you realize that those who report arthritis as a symptom are many times more likely to report other diseases as well. Especially those related to the heart and lungs.

Arthritis may be only an early sign of generalized deterioration of the person as a whole. That's what I've repeatedly found; a person with a major disease such as diabetes or rheumatoid arthritis usually has several other, apparently unrelated, health problems. It looks to me suspiciously like a generalized degradation of health.

ARTHRITIS AS A SYMPTOM OF POOR HEALTH

Is there any evidence that being arthritic relates to poor health? Yes.

The Journal of Rheumatology published an article in February 1995 which maintained the connection. The Rochester Epidemiology Project and survey reported that people with osteoarthritis incur substantially more medical costs, not only for arthritis care, but also for the care of neurological, gastrointestinal, cardiac, and respiratory conditions as compared to non-arthritics. This data also demonstrated important and statistically significantly higher levels of work disability among people with osteoarthritis compared to their age and sex-adjusted peers without arthritis, but from the same community.

In Canada as in the US the most frequently reported reason for long term disability is both major types of arthritis, osteoarthritis being the most common. Almost one out of every 5 residents of Ontario, Canada who sought medical attention in 1995 listed arthritis as an important symptom. An appreciable proportion of this group used health care resources and continued to do so over the long duration of the condition. . . which basically meant until they died. Long-term disability was accompanied by a substantial effect on daily life.

They had:
>Troubles with mobility.
A lack of independence.
Difficulty with everyday living activities.
Social isolation.
Curtailment of leisure.
Less employment.
Lower incomes.

The exact same conditions exist with other chronic diseases such as fibromyalgia. To a lesser degree we might also include asthma and the gastrointestinal complaints like irritable bowel.

Arthritis can change an older person's life to that of a complete invalid. Simple tasks that one had taken for granted become difficult and exasperating.

Tasks like:
>Raising the arms for something in a higher cabinet.
Lifting common objects that were easy before.
Walking 1 or 2 blocks to visit a neighbor or market.
Bathing or showering.
Climbing, even as little as 10 steps.
Pain while grasping an object like a needle or a spoon.
Getting in or out of bed.
Dressing.
Using the toilet.
Preparing meals.
Doing personal shopping.
Doing heavy or even light housework.

These tasks seem so simple, and they should be, but not for those afflicted with arthritis or similar diseases.

OSTEOARTHRITIS

There are 500,000 new cases each year, and these cases are just the ones that get reported.

Osteoarthritis is responsible for 46 million physician visits a year, and 68 million lost work days a year. 85% of Americans have it by age 65.

Osteoarthritis is a profound disease that cripples but does not kill. It's not supposed to be an inflammatory disease, yet most say there must be some inflammation. Somewhat like rheumatoid arthritis, there is pain, restriction of joint movements, and loss of strength in the limbs.

SHIRLEY

A 50-year-old female with a family history of arthritis, Shirley had herself become a victim for several years. She complained of severe pain in both shoulders. Both hands were swollen and painful. There was limited mobility of her fingers with the signs of some inflammation. Her doctor had diagnosed her as having osteoarthritis because her laboratory tests did not indicate it was rheumatoid. He prescribed the usual non-steroidal anti-inflammatories, which helped, but it left her feeling abnormal.

3 days after she started *CMO* she began to feel some relief. The pain left first, then the mobility of her fingers increased. Finally the swelling started to abate. When she felt her fingers were about back to normal, she had her rings resized. The swellings had come on so gradually, she had not noticed just how much they had deformed her fingers.

She had always enjoyed skiing but stopped years ago because of the arthritis. The improvements reactivated her interests so she made her arrangements and went to the mountains. To her delight she was able to ski with no difficulty from her shoulders or hands. As of this writing she has not had to repeat the *CMO* treatments.

RUBY

This religious lady had suffered from severe osteoarthritis for over 10 years. Now 63, she woke every morning to agonizing pain and stiffness. Gradually, she had stopped all but the most simple chores. As an active Seventh Day Adventist, she had resisted using medications, utilizing, instead, avoidance of the nightshades and other triggering foods.

She was still debating what to do when she heard about *CMO* and decided to give it a try. The pain and stiffness disappeared within 10 days, but the range of movements of her joints have taken longer. She uses the joints to their full limits as often as she can but is still working on it. Things are still in their improvement stages for her, but the pain and swelling has not returned.

BERTHA

This is a 78-year-old female with diagnosed osteoarthritis and macular degeneration. She had laser surgery and a hip replacement in the last year. For as long as she could remember she had been taking anti-inflammatory drugs for her gradually worsening joints. Her symptoms were the same as everyone with arthritis: pain, swelling and limited movements.

It took her almost a month to notice any improvements but she was grateful when they came. Gradually, she was able to discontinue her medications. It took even more time for her to readjust to the new mobility. She was so used to staying at home and doing nothing, her new freedom was scary. Not being a quitter, she made a special effort to retrain herself to independence, relying less on people, as she had become accustomed to doing.

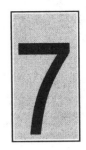

RHEUMATOID ARTHRITIS

What can you say about a disease that makes your life a living hell—then kills you. If you have rheumatoid arthritis you may live longer than a cancer patient, but you may wish you hadn't. Rheumatoid arthritis is a disease that steadily advances. As it worsens, the medications begin to fail, then stronger and more toxic drugs are necessary. The side effects of these drugs will begin to ruin your health, and your quality of life will ebb away.

RHEUMATOID ARTHRITIS AS YOU GET OLDER

This will not come as good news, but rheumatoid arthritis is one of those things we have to worry about as we get older. Why? Because rheumatoid arthritis becomes more common as a population ages; especially as the group passes 60. Even worse. . . rheumatoid arthritis, at this age, seems to be more severe and more disabling than that which strikes the youngster.

The cartilage and bone of joints are highly dynamic

tissues; during disease they speed up even more: poorly integrated cells slough off along with the discarded cells to gum up the joint and the whole place is flooded with white blood cells (leukocytes)—everything gets hot, bloated and painful.

Now that we can expect to live longer, our chances of acquiring rheumatoid arthritis are better than ever.

DOES ARTHRITIS AND ILL HEALTH GO TOGETHER?

In study after study, ailments related to arthritis seem common. In psoriatic arthritis, for example, doctors frequently find subclinical gut inflammation. So, which came first, the gut problem or the arthritis? No one can say.

One of the problems that occurs when we use cortisone to treat rheumatoid arthritis is the problem of bone thinning and fractures. This results in vertebral deformities because of the thinning. Fifty eight percent of women receiving long-term cortisone suffer this tragedy. Women are led into these disasters as lambs to the slaughter by doctors who are shortsighted and narrow-minded. "Just keep the line moving, please, and never mind tomorrow." And, "We'll worry about that when it gets here." When tomorrow brings the disaster, and we suddenly realize we have a non-reversible deformity, what do we hear? "Well, you should have expected such things." Of course, we never dreamed such a thing would happen to us. The doctor knew, but he wouldn't tell us, he was just too busy.

Thank God there are alternatives.

Now, thanks to *CMO*, you can toss away your cane, crutches and wheelchairs because there is a good chance you won't need them any more. . . and, oh yes, go ahead and make arrangements for those clogging lessons you've been putting off.

WINDY

When I first saw Windy she had endured rheumatoid arthritis for 10 years and was suffering from all of the deformities that are typical of patients with the more severe types. She had a rheumatoid factor of 270 and x-ray confirmation of multiple joint involvement. And, of course, she had all of the symptoms, including the fear of being touched. Everything hurt, day and night, so she got very little quality sleep.

She could raise her arms to a horizontal level, but no higher: she could barely squat. All of her fingers were frozen and malaligned, and her knuckles were overgrown, raised, hard, hot and extremely tender. She complained of extreme fatigue and depression.

Windy took her **CMO** twice daily and noticed nothing different for the first 24 hours. On the morning of the third day she awoke rested for the first time in years, and realized that she had slept through the night without tossing and turning from pain. She also noticed that there was a definite change in her sense of tightness and stiffness. Although her frozen joints never flexed, everything moved easier and smoother: she slipped out of bed without the uncertain stiffness. She felt around and all of the painful spots were gone.

Her hands, which were normally cold, felt warm for the first time, she remembered. During the day she noticed about a 10% overall relief of pain as compared to prior days.

By the fourth day she felt much more flexible. The index fingers of both hands actually flexed for the first time in years. She was able to squat a little deeper and could bounce up and down without pain.

At the end of a week she was 100% free of pain most of the time and, of course, sleeping much better. Her depression and fatigue were totally gone. She was now able to raise her arms about 15% higher than before and squat deeper. Unfortunately, her fingers were not closing as fast as we had hoped for, but all of the swelling around her joints was gone.

During the third week she had a return of pain in her left hip, but nowhere else. Everything else seemed to continue to improve.

After 4 weeks she could raise her right arm almost vertical and her left arm at about a 45 degree angle. She could squat almost to the floor. Her hip pain was gone and she was ready to have new laboratory tests and new x-rays of her joints.

KEN

Ken is 72 years old and was confined to a wheelchair for two years because of rheumatoid arthritis. He has had the disease for over 11 years, with it steadily progressing until he was reduced to a wheelchair. The joint pains were so intense that he needed pain medication almost constantly. He had the usual morning stiffness which took hours to work out.

Gold had not helped and he had side effects to methotrexate, so he was still on NSAIDs and with cortisone occasionally.

His most difficult symptoms were in his lower extremities. His hips, knees and ankles. Ken had profound fatigue and depression, part of which may have been due to his finding out he was beginning to have diabetes and hypertension.

CMO put Ken back on his feet. He couldn't run or dance but he could move right along on his own. He was also still taking an aspirin once in a while, but 90% of his pains were gone. The swellings around the joints in his knees and ankles are gone too.

PAUL

Paul was X-ray and laboratory positive for rheumatoid

arthritis. At age 61 he was using a walker after only 4 years with the disease. For him the problems were mostly in his back and hips. He needed pain medications but fought off using them most of the time almost as an attempt to deny he was sick. From time to time he would have almost a roving myalgia along with severe fatigue.

He started *CMO* and within a week was able to walk without his support. His recovery was fairly rapid considering the severity of his symptoms. Almost all of his symptoms are gone now, although he still has some residual rigidity. I said rigidity, not stiffness because, even though the disease has passed, it's left some structural damage in its wake, which is probably permanent.

ELIZABETH

A 45-year-old female was given the bad news by her physician, "The tests show you have rheumatoid arthritis." For 7 months she had felt it coming on but had denied it as long as she could. Now she found herself almost unable to leave her bed in the morning because of the stiffness and pain. Thinking it would just be a matter of serious intent she hired a personal trainer to work out the stiffness. It took only one session for her to realize this was a dream. Her muscle strength had declined so much she was unable to hold even a 5-pound weight.

Soon afterwards she required a wheelchair to move around, and now she found herself spending days at a time in bed. Her hands were almost useless by this time. She saw her physician, but was apparently undermedicated.

CMO was only slightly helpful during the first two weeks. It was during the second series that she noticed the most improvement.

She now works out in a gym without pain or incident. She does not have early morning stiffness and pain, and she has resumed her normal life. Now she looks back at it as a nightmare that has come and gone. It came on so rapidly it was frightening, but it left with even greater speed, thanks to the magic of *CMO*.

VANCE

An electrician in his mid 30's was diagnosed as having the beginnings of rheumatoid arthritis. Over a two year period his life took a steady downhill course. Each day he walked around in pain. It seemed like everything hurt: his ankles, knees, hips, shoulders, back and hands. The job was getting harder, and he was now taking more sick days. Before he went to work each day he had to run warm water over his hands to unstiffen and loosen them.

He dreaded the mornings because it took so long to loosen up, and it was painful to do so. 4 hours into the job and he was completely miserable. It was difficult to hold things, especially heavy things, and this made him clumsy and awkward.

In addition to medications he had attempted to adjust his diet and was taking every supplement he had read about that would reverse his arthritis. None worked. He gave up weekend hiking early on, but now the worry wasn't what to do on weekends, it was what to do if he couldn't work anymore.

His blood work indicated rheumatoid arthritis.

It took several weeks of urging to get him on *CMO*, and it was difficult to keep him on it because he didn't respond early on. At the end of the second week he expressed discouragement and wanted to stop, believing that he was going to be one of the few who do not benefit from *CMO.*

Fortunately, he gave in and tried it a few more days. He first noticed something when he was warming his hands under the warm water. It took less time to get them loose. Then he noticed they weren't as stiff or as painful when he awoke. He climbed a ladder one day without difficulty and that was the time when he decided that he was responding and he admitted it to himself.

By the sixth week he had no morning pains at all. From then on all of the symptoms gradually diminished. On his next physician visit his sedimentation rate (a test that indicates a chronic inflammation) had returned to normal. He had virtually no symptoms, so his medications were discontinued. His doctor said he was going into remission, but not to worry, it would all come back. The electrician doesn't think so.

MORE ON FISH OIL AND RHEUMATOID ARTHRITIS

Let's look at another study. An article in the 1995 Scandinavian Journal of Rheumatology stated there was significant reduction in the usage of anti-inflammatory drugs after three months of fish oil.

Fish oil can even be injected, but it must first be emulsified. The authors of an article in the June 92 issue of the Proceedings of the Society for Experimental Biology and Medicine noted that there are times when we cannot wait for the slow process and we need the immediate benefits of *fish oil*. Such a situation might occur in an acute rejection of grafts. When n-3 fish oil was injected in animals under similar stress there was major suppression of the beginning of the inflammatory process.

FISH OIL IMPROVES LABORATORY TESTS

It's been reported that laboratory tests improve significantly after the use of fish oil. Levels of Interleukin (an inflammatory producer) also dropped significantly after 12 weeks on the fish oil supplements.

Another report from the Annals of the Rheumatic Disease

(July 1992) found that sedimentary rates dropped in 10 patients treated with fish oil, and white blood cell activity declined significantly too. This is very important because part of the problem with rheumatoid arthritis, according to the Journal of Leukocyte Biology (1994), is that there are too many white blood cells. White blood cells are known to enter the joints in great numbers, spewing huge amounts of free radicals that eat away at the tissues and create ugly deformities. The essential fatty acids that are found in fish oil can be seen suppressing T lymphocytes (one type of white blood cell) by as much as 80%.

I am particularly sensitive to the fact that *CMO* is most closely related to fish oil. *CMO* might be considered a type of fish oil since it is known to come from the sperm whale. I make this point because other oils, including the other essential fatty acids like flax and evening primrose don't have the same effectiveness as fish oil.

It is pretty well accepted that flax seed oil is not as effective as fish oil on arthritis. Evening primrose oil may make it worse.

Even olive oil has been considered therapeutic, in fact, olive oil was compared to fish oil in an experiment published in the June 94 issue of Arthritis and Rheumatism. The conclusion was that olive oil had no benefit to rheumatoid arthritis, but fish oil significantly improved the patients.

VEGGIE DIET

Can a diet improve fish oils effectiveness? Yes. . . the veggie diet.

It is known that the vegetarian diet has a lower percent of arachidonic acid (the inflammatory fatty acid). At the same time, though, it does not have a higher percent of n-3s (anti-inflammatory fatty acids). But merely lowering the amount of arachidonic acid in the diet is greatly helpful, and then when fish oil is added it makes a great difference. This appeared in the German publication Zeitschrift fur Rheumatologie (Sept.) 1993.

VITAMIN E AND FISH OIL

Another thing that enhanced fish oil was Vitamin E. It doesn't take much. 200 or 400 units is more than enough.

DIET FACTORS IN RHEUMATOID ARTHRITIS

The German Journal Zeitschrift fur Rheumatologie, May 1993, said that foods high in saturated fats predispose to osteoarthritis. It agreed that fish oil supplements greatly help the diet in this disease. Then the authors said that sugar predisposes to osteoarthritis, and promotes the development of degenerative joint disease in predisposed mice.

PSORIATIC ARTHRITIS

Patients with psoriatic arthritis may have other problems as well as those we've already covered. An article in the Journal of Rheumatology 1995, found 25 patients to have less selenium, less omega 6 EFAs, and increased copper. This study supports the view that an abnormal fatty acid pattern might be a particular metabolic modification involved or associated with the patho-genesis of rheumatoid arthritis.

As you can see, the fatty acid disturbances found in all types of arthritis pop up endlessly. Oils play a major role in the disease and they play a major role in its cure.

THE PROTOCOL FOR ARTHRITIS

The *CMO* protocol for the treatment of arthritis is very simple.

Take three 75mg capsules of CETYL MYRISTOLEATE twice a day on an empty stomach for 8 days, then stop.

No capsules for the next 8 days, then resume three capsules daily till through. (Save 8 capsules for back-up).

One does NOT have to diet while taking **CMO**, but I'm including the diet because I think it improves the chances that **CMO** will survive digestion, by removing foods that may undermine **CMO**'s survival.

A DIET FOR THE TWO WEEKS OF THE PROGRAM

1. NO ALCOHOL DURING THIS PERIOD. IN FACT, YOU SHOULDN'T HAVE ANY FOR A FEW DAYS BEFORE STARTING THE PROGRAM.
2. NO CHOCOLATE DURING THIS PERIOD OF TIME.
3. NO CAFFEINE DURING THIS THREE WEEK TREATMENT PERIOD (NO COFFEE, TEA, COLAS, DRINKS OR FOOD OR FOOD SUPPLEMENTS, LIKE HERBS WHICH CONTAIN CAFFEINE).
4. EAT A MODIFIED VEGETARIAN DIET WITH LESS SUGAR AND SATURATED FATS. (DO NOT EAT CANDY OR USE SUGAR OTHER THAN FRUITS).
5. AVOID SATURATED AND RANCID FATS. SALAD OILS AND ESSENTIAL FATTY ACIDS ARE ALL RIGHT.

MEDICATIONS

NO STEROIDS FOR 5 DAYS BEFORE THE TREATMENT AND UNTIL 5 DAYS AFTER THE TREATMENT. DO NOT DISCONTINUE STEROIDS IN CASES WHERE THEY ARE CRITICAL FOR SYMPTOM CONTROL. YOU MAY CONTINUE ANY OF YOUR OTHER DRUGS FOR ARTHRITIS AS WELL AS OTHER AILMENTS.

NOTE: I STRONGLY ADVISE ANYONE USING THIS PROGRAM TO DO IT UNDER THE SUPERVISION OF A PHYSICIAN.

FINAL THOUGHTS

I, and other doctors who use **CMO**, have confirmed **CMO**'s ability to reverse the symptoms of arthritis. It's rare to see an arthritic resist *CMO's* effects, and what a pleasure it is when a difficult case really comes around.

A rather bleak future can be redrawn, now that we have *CMO.*

Rheumatoid arthritis, more than almost all other disease, is a symptom of generalized poor health. Even if the victim's health was normal at the start, it changes. The steady strain of a severe inflammation erodes away all prior health.

The opposite is true, too. As one's health declines through aging, the chances of acquiring rheumatoid arthritis go up.

Deterioration of heart muscle, in this case the so-called "silent heart disease", is one of the most serious and dangerous of these unseen effects of poor health.

And then there is the problem with the medicines. I'm not talking about side effects, I'm talking about the problem of drugs becoming less and less effective over time. Called tachyphylaxis, the declining effectiveness of the drugs is a big handicap to doctors who have to treat chronic diseases. What it means is that doctors have to periodically increase the strength of the current medicines, or switch to stronger medicines. . . either of which is likely to cause toxicity.

Rheumatic disease, as it advances, has an enormous impact on quality of life. All relationships become strained; marriages, romances, family ties and obligations.

The rheumatoid arthritic dreads being touched. This feeling is so painful, even relatives have to respect this. Pain from being touched often continues even when the patient is on methotrexate, a strong anti-inflammatory drug.

CMO quickly removes the pain of being touched in every case that I have seen or heard of.

YOU need to know that drug-free pain relief can be as little as *one week away.*

Recovering full joint movement may take longer, but it will

happen. From what I have observed, the patients who carefully exercise their joints, after they are no longer inflamed, recover their range of motion more rapidly, so I encourage it. This is shocking to patients who have been told not to exercise.

There are cases in which **CMO** has softened the deformities. It usually takes a while, because remolding tissue is a lengthy process. This possibility while small should bring hope to many whose deformities are almost too ugly to look at, and who have had to stay in hiding for years.

What does it feel like to be a recovering arthritic? What should you expect now? It's been my experience that the change is so rapid you won't believe you are well, even after you no longer have symptoms.

Watching the recovered arthritic is like watching a blind man with new eyes. Some won't try things because they believe they can't do them.

<u>It will take a long time for you to realize how much you have had to give up because of the arthritis.</u>

You may be afraid to discontinue the medicines you no longer need when the symptoms are gone—talk to your doctor about it.

Activities you've learned to avoid need to be tried. You may have to push yourself to try something as simple as reaching up for things, or using individual fingers instead of clutching things with two frozen "lobster" claws. From now on, it's use it or lose it.

I encourage you to keep a diary so you can fully appreciate how rapidly the changes are coming.

Next comes the worry about arthritis returning. Experience has shown that in some, it may. . . and as early as a few months. . . a joint pain. . . a sore spot. . . nothing big, but just an early warning. But now, all you have to do to eliminate the problem is to take a few capsules of *CMO*, and the symptoms usually disappear like magic.

In working with arthritic patients I've often observed that a single capsule is more than enough to remove returning symptoms in the majority of cases. Some people are more fortunate than others: one course of *CMO* is enough—they never experience arthritis again.

You may have been so damaged by their disease you still require knee or joint replacements. *CMO* can't change this. *CMO* can eliminate the disease, but it can't undo the damage. You may need to go forward with surgical repairs.

SUPPORTIVE NUTRIENTS FOR *CMO*

When it comes to arthritis and *CMO* I tell my patients to use three excellent supporting nutrients. First: three 1000 mg capsules of fish oil daily along with a tablespoonful of flax seed oil twice a day. Don't worry it won't have a negative effect on your weight. It increases your metabolic efficiency to a point where you might even lose weight.

Second, I use rheumatoid forte (collagen type 2), and third I suggest a special sulfur tablet called Biomax from the GYN 800-526-3030. KNOLLWOOD HAS *CMO* 800-249-7816.

SPECIAL NOTE

If your physician tests your rheumatoid factor while you are on *CMO*, or soon after you have been on it, *the results may be highly elevated.* Please note that these factors are rising at the same time your symptoms are disappearing. This does not mean your disease is going underground, instead it means your defenses are growing enormously. Many scientists believe this plasma factor is a positive sign your body is fighting back, and the higher the better. Your sed rate on the other hand may return to normal.

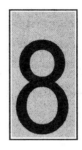

MUSCULO-SKELETAL DISEASES

THE PARA-RHEUMATIC DISORDERS OF THE MUSCULO-SKELETAL SYSTEM

In this section, I'll be talking about diseases that have often been called *soft tissue rheum atism:* chronically painful muscles, fascia and tendons. Usually they're caused by old traumas or by years of endless small traumas. I'll talk a little about fibromyalgia too.

My experience is that this musculo-skeletal group of diseases responds about as well to **CMO** as do the arthritics.

RECENT TRAUMAS: AN EXCEPTION

If you have recently turned a knee or sprained an ankle don't bother with **CMO**. I can tell you up front, **CMO** will probably not help you. New injuries rarely respond to **CMO** because too little time has passed for there to be a depletion of EFAs. Healthy people have adequate reserves of EFAs. In order for the EFAs to become depleted the injury has to have remained chronically inflamed for a sufficient period of time.

You could try *CMO*, of course. It won't hurt you, but it's unlikely to do you any good. I've tried *CMO* under these circumstances and so have other doctors. The consensus of opinion is that *CMO* is seldom useful for new traumas.

Recall my prior statements on this: *CMO* will help if the problem can be fixed by the use of fatty acids, *BUT* the EFAs must have been deficient or imbalanced to start with.

It is true that *CMO* suppresses inflammations, but all inflammations are not the same. A new inflammation has different dynamics than a chronic one. A new inflammation has not developed autoimmune components yet, nor has there been time enough to develop an EFA deficiency—the necessary conditions for *CMO* to work.

PAINFUL EXTREMITIES

LEE

Lee's a middle aged insurance salesman who had been complaining to his wife about the pain in his feet for five years. His feet looked normal. There were no deformities, bunions, corns, spurs or signs of tendonitis, bursitis or capsulitis. His feet had color and warmth, so the circulation looked adequate. A bad choice of shoes could have been the source of his pains, but in Lee's case that wasn't true.

Lee was on his feet too often, we decided. He, like truck drivers and others whose feet are important to their work, develop pains from constant foot action—it's an occupational hazard.

The pains in Lee's feet disappeared in three days, removed by *CMO*. At my insistence, he stayed on *CMO* for another 10 days to build up adequate reserves. Unlike a medicine, *CMO* satisfies something the body needs. Without *CMO* we are susceptible to chronic disease, especially musculo-skeletal diseases: therefore, it's good to have extra for any upcoming needs.

Women complain of feet pains as often as men. I don't have to tell you why, you're way ahead of me on this one: designer shoes. Every part of the foot can hurt from a beautiful pair of fashion statements.

Digital (toe) disorders most frequently result from poor shoe choices. *CMO* removes the pain, but not for long if you insist on wearing the same type shoes. The pain will come back if you continue the activity that caused the problem.

CMO can help some deformities of the feet. There is a condition called hallux valgus, for example, that may be helped. Hallux valgus is a condition where the big toe turns abruptly to the side, often sliding under the next toe causing it to develop into a hammer toe. *CMO* can reduce pain and loosen joints to improve the potential of orthotic treatments.

Would you believe that 4 million people have pes plano valgus? That's flat feet.

The flatfooted person tries to compensate for the problem by using another part of the foot for support during walking. This can strain adjacent areas, causing painful feet.

CMO can lower the pains in the adjacent areas of the feet which are caused by the difficulty in walking, but it can't repair the broken tendons.

The heel is another site for foot trauma. As you take a step when you walk, tendons slide back and forth under the heel bone. This constant friction can cause spur formations. One can develop sore spots on the heels that never seem to go away, even without the spur formations. *CMO* can help.

LINDA

Linda, a 47-year-old female, was worried about her hands. The thumbs and fingers of both hands were stiff and hurting when she tried to make a fist, which meant that every time she used her hands they hurt afterwards.

Her feet were even worse—they hurt all the time.

She used a lot of aspirin for pain. Then she discovered that steam baths relieved the foot pains. Most of the cramps came out in the hot steam, so she used the baths as often as she could.

Linda tried to make the best of it. She worked hard to develop a good attitude about the whole thing since she knew she would never be free of the problem.

But something happened!

As she walked around her house one morning she noticed her feet had stopped hurting, it was on the third day of *CMO.* She continued taking *CMO* for the next week, then stopped. The foot pains were gone.

Two months later she began to feel the pains returning to her feet and the stiffness returning to her hands. After two days of *CMO,* the pain and stiffness left again. A month later the pains started once more. This time she took *CMO* for 8 days. Once again the pains and stiffness disappeared—for good.

It's been a year and a half and she hasn't had further problems. She can make a fist now without pain. Her fingers move through about 95% of their normal range of motion.

The pain may or may not return. It doesn't matter, because she knows what to do about it if it does.

A good rule of thumb is if the problem is old and has an arthritic feel about it, or if it seems to be an "all worn out" type of pain, then *CMO* has a better chance of working.

BURSITIS, TENDONITIS, MYOSITIS, CAPSULITIS, CARPAL TUNNEL

Any joint or muscle in a limb can become chronically inflamed, sore and hard to move. There are plenty of drugs available for these conditions, of course, but it is surprising how many people find them undesirable and less than effective. The drugs rarely stop the disease: mainly they provide a little symptom relief.

We can partially blame the patient for creating this chronic condition. People who do not fully comply with their doctor's request that they not use the affected joint until the joint has had time to heal, cause themselves permanent problems. By ignoring good advice, patients convert acute conditions into chronic ones.

Let's look at a group of people with musculo-skeletal problems.

RON

Ron was a skier. And when he wasn't skiing he was golfing. He decided to drive up to mammoth last winter and ski. Mammoth Mountain is a ski haven on the eastern slopes of California's Sierra Nevada Mountains. It's an extremely cold place in the middle of winter. Boy, is it cold! If you're not dressed properly, the cold can be brutal. Ron loved the cold and usually did well in it. But on the first morning of this trip he noticed some unusual stiffness in his hands, and occasional finger pains as he moved up the ski lift.

After a half day on the slopes he found it almost impossible to control his ski poles. His hands were hurting so bad there was no fun in what he was doing. Ron decided to cut his trip short, he came home disappointed.

The warm sun over his Southern California home enticed

him into some golf. He started his game and a half hour later began to have the same trouble. His hands throbbed so much after hitting a few balls that he was not able to finish 18 holes. As soon as he reached home he had his physician call in a prescription for pain medication.

Thinking back, he discovered that his problem had really been coming on for some time. As men often do, he had discounted some prior episodes of stiffness in his hands, thinking it was probably soreness from extra use.

He took his **CMO** for 12 days and the pains disappeared completely, and there was no residual stiffness or pain in his hands or fingers. He admits he still has a few small twinges when he plays golf, but they are too minor to mention, and they don't affect his game. And Ron has skied once since he took **CMO**, without experiencing difficulties.

ALEX

A 58-year-old male, Alex had a bad knee. He often slept in his recliner because of it. Lying in bed flat caused the knee to hurt, keeping him awake.

His knee injury came about during his college football days when his knee was repeatedly battered. That same knee was reinjured at work a few years later and it eventually required three knee operations.

The surgeries did not solve his pain problem, though. He was still taking 12 ibuprofen a day and that was not enough, according to him. In spite of the medications, he had developed arthritis in the joint.

His knee pain disappeared overnight after taking 3 capsules of **CMO** at bedtime. He took 4 capsules a day for two more weeks, then stopped. He says his knee gets sore once in a while after he overexerts, but it goes away with one aspirin.

Except for occasional soreness he's essentially pain free. After a year he still hasn't had to use **CMO** again.

RUTH

Just after Ruth's sixtieth birthday she fell down and injured her hip. For a full year she suffered almost constant pain. She refused medicines from her physician, and instead tried various methods of natural healing. Nothing she tried made any difference. She said she was about to give in and make a doctor's appointment for a prescription when she had second thoughts, and decided to give natural healing one last chance.

Fortunately for her, **CMO** had just become available. She took 4 capsules a day for the first 5 days without any relief and had decided that it was not going to work. Discouraged, she made her doctor's appointment. But when she woke up on the sixth morning she noticed less pain. She restarted the **CMO** and the next morning there was even less pain. And so it went until the 12th day when she awoke pain free.

You must have noticed that the severity of the disease does not determine the rapidity of improvement. I have seen minor problems respond slowly over weeks, while more serious diseases improve almost overnight. I'm sure the degree of response is related to the degree of EFA deficiency more than anything else. This would be entirely reasonable since a serious disease would be more stressful on the body, which would seriously depress the available EFAs.

PAUL

A physician who was injured in an automobile accident 10 years back was left with a pronounced limp in his left leg. He had to swing his leg out to the side in order to walk. During the last few years he noticed that his hip and affected leg were developing arthritic-like pains.

He placed himself on *CMO* shortly after he heard about it. On the third day he was pain free in both the hip and the leg. He says his activities have not changed, he is doing nothing different, yet he has not had to use *CMO* again.

LISA

Lisa, an accountant in Southern California, had bilateral knee problems from the age of 8, when she was struck by a car. From the time of her accident until she took *CMO,* her knees got steadily worse, according to her. The main knee symptoms were: pain, stiffness and swelling.

She used the standard 4 capsules of *CMO* daily, for 15 days, and the symptoms slowly disappeared. The first time she really appreciated what was happening was when she tried some heels on and wore them for the first time in 6 years.

She accepted an invitation to a rock concert a few days later. There, she found a dance floor crowded with people.

Feeling good, and throwing caution to the wind, she decided to *give it a try.* Impulsively, she jumped up from her table and dove into the crowd on the dance floor. She bounced up and down and twisted around with the rest of them. . . for three hours. Afterwards, she was sore for several days but that went away, never to return. She reports never having to take *CMO* again.

SAM

Sam is a computer kind of guy. He makes his living on it and needs nimble fingers. Unfortunately, his fingers have been slowly locking up on him due to a gradually developing osteoarthritis. It had gotten to the point where he wasn't able to make a fist with either hand. His fingers closed no more than 15% of their normal range. This made him look like he was about to catch a basketball all the time.

His fingers hurt too. Especially if he used them extensively—and he needed them for his income. He was facing a crisis. There had to be some radical improvements soon or he would have to face a career change, a not-too-happy situation when you're in your early fifties.

I started Sam on **CMO** and in three weeks his left hand was 90% better and his right hand, while improved by 25%, was not nearly where he needed it. Fortunately, his pains were almost all gone. We repeated the treatment with a higher dose and got the changes in the right hand that he needed.

Sam is still a computer kind of guy.

MICHAEL

This chiropractor injured the rotator cuff in his right shoulder. Like most such injuries, it got better but never really went away. And while he was not conscious of his shoulder most of the time, any unusual movement would quickly remind him he hadn't gotten over the injury.

He liked to mow his own lawn, but couldn't because of the pain it inflicted. Changes in the weather would cause his shoulder to ache. During sleep, if he turned onto his right side, the pain would wake him. After two years of repeated aggravation he noticed the pain was becoming continual. It had gotten so that now he could feel low-grade pains all the time.

He began taking two capsules of **CMO** twice a day. He kept a chart on himself and recorded zero pain on the second day. He began sleeping through the night, which meant he was occasionally on his right side with no pain. Two weeks after he finished his **CMO** he took his wife to a concert, and while listening to the music, he kept his right arm around his wife's shoulders for over an hour and a half. This was an unconscious and spontaneous action on his part, but as they left his wife mentioned it to him. He moved his arm throughout its full range of motion and could find no position which caused pain.

PAT

Pat is a mailman who developed bilaterial carpal tunnel syndrome. Undoubtedly the wrist inflammations came about as a result of his occupation. The first time he noticed his wrist bothering him was when he was pushing a mail cart at the post office, and from there it seemed like the inflammation worsened over several years. It hurt enough for him to see a chiropractor who made the diagnosis of carpal tunnel syndrome.

The treatments were unsuccessful and his wife was finally down to wrapping his wrists with Ace bandages before he left for work each day. If she hadn't, he wouldn't have been able to drive his route.

The wrist pains, he said, disappeared after taking *CMO* for two weeks.

It's now been 6 months with no return of the symptoms.

Pat sacks mail, stuffs post boxes, drives his vehicle, pushes carts and uses his wrists. He does all this without any signs of pain, discomfort, or restriction of movement.

CHRISTY

Christy told me about her TMJ problem in the middle of our weight maintenance session. We were planning her long-term weight control strategy now that she was no longer overweight. She hadn't mentioned her jaw before because she didn't realize I was able to help.

Her trouble began in 1981 while she was working in Albuquerque, New Mexico. She has no memory of how it started: all she can remember is that it came on fast. Her earliest vision was her hand pressed against a cheek.

She saw a chiropractor, and he manipulated her jaw, which she thinks probably made it worse. Next, she visited a neurosurgeon who offered her pain medications.

She was in a heavy romance at the time, which budded eventually into a marriage. But, she said, it did not get off to a good start. She spent her wedding night pacing up and down the bridal suite with two packs of ice pressed against her jaws.

Her next professional helper was a dentist. She remembers having a liquid injected into the joints and X-rays taken. Her dentist then constructed a splint, which she wore 24 hours a day. The pain gradually subsided but the misalignment did not really change. From then until January 1996 she saw a number of other dentists specializing in TMJ, with little benefit. Christy said the pains always came and went, but never really stabilized.

In February of 1996 a dentist put a crown on a tooth in her lower left jaw. The placement completely destabilized her jaw alignment and she experienced pains exceeding anything she had ever felt before.

Prior to our conversation she had been taking 9 advil a day as well as a number of prescription codeine tablets. The nocturnal pains kept her tossing: there was no such thing as sleep.

This turn of events was extremely unfortunate, because her occupation required her to use her jaw constantly: she was an airline representative.

Desperate, Christy sought the help of an acupuncturist, and stuck it out for four sessions. This in spite of the fact the treatments seemed to be making it worse. She developed nausea and weakness, including a general sense of malaise.

I immediately placed her on **CMO.**

She called me back later in the day to say that her pains were subsiding, and the next day she reported an 80% relief in symptoms, especially pain. *CMO* is a mood elevator, she said she noticed that as well.

JACK

Jack is a 37-year-old policeman with an addiction for athletic activities, including practicing the triathlon. He especially loves to run. However, Jack has one big problem—he has bad knees. Nevertheless, his love for running is so great that he packs his knees in ice before and after runs so he can get through the run. He's had cortisone shots, but they were painful and short-lived. Shark cartilage was slightly helpful, but not much better than most of the other things he had tried.

In the spring of 1996, Jack entered the marathon between Baker, California and Las Vegas, Nevada. That's a 90-mile stretch of the driest desert you've ever seen. Each runner, in the race carries a baton, runs 5 miles, then passes it on. Jack was told he would be the starter, running up the steep incline out of Baker.

He was calculating the pounds of ice required for the race when a friend suggested *CMO.*

Jack took the *CMO* several weeks before the race, not really expecting much. To his surprise and relief, it worked. He was pain free for the first time in years. In spite of his improvements he brought the ice for the race anyway, just in case.

Just before the race, Jack limbered up on the asphalt highway in the early morning sun, glancing now and then at the hill he was going up—pain or no pain.

The gun sounded and he started his uphill run, wondering how long it would be before the pains cut in as they had in the past. He waited and he waited, but it didn't happen. He was racing like the wind, as if his knees were greased.

Inside he was screaming with excitement, but in the far recesses of his mind there was another worry. The uphill part of the race wasn't the hard part. There was a steep downhill section. That was the part he dreaded. Downhill running causes tremendous joint trauma as the bones slam together with each step.

Jack was almost to the top without pain, still moving easily. He raced up over the long curve, crested, then started the descent. He waited, his mind alert for the first twinges, the prickles, the sharp jabs—nothing! He couldn't believe what was happening, he *STILL* doesn't believe what happened.

At the end of five pain-free miles, Jack passed the baton. He rested a while then climbed into his transportation. He was being driven to Las Vegas to be there when the race finished. On the way, he waited for the throbbing to begin, keeping his ice close by—he never used it.

Weeks later, Jack was still waiting for the throbbing to begin. . . it hasn't. He shakes his head in amazement every time he relates the story.

REMEDIES FOR LEG AND FOOD CRAMPS

CMO will probably take care of all of your old aches and pains but if you develop any new aches or pains then here's some things I have used. I recommend they apply ten drops of an over-the-counter cold medicine, and rub it in to the affected area slowly. Robitussin (guaifenesin) is the only one that works virtually every time. Some people need more than ten drops to work out the soreness.

Some of my athletic patients turned me on to a spray called "Kool and Fit". Bicyclists use this spray before, and during marathons. They spray it onto the affected calf or thigh muscle and let it evaporate. It can be effective on any painful area. I have found it to be sleep inducing also, just a single drop under the chin does the job.

CARRIE

The last case is a 42-year-old female who was accidentally shot by a 9mm hollow point bullet on November 2, 1995. The bullet tore through her left arm, leaving massive damage and entered her left chest. Steel fragments spread through her arm, chest and abdomen. She still carries these fragments, many were not removed because of the hazards of surgery.

After her surgery and acute phase she was assigned to physiotherapy. One of the first problems her therapist faced was the restoration of circulation to the left arm. The major obstruction was a huge band of edema in her left shoulder, including the axillary area. The surgical incision was not healing as fast as was desirable either. It looked red and inflamed and swollen.

Without her doctor's knowledge she began using *CMO*. She needed a miracle, a few side effects were of no concern.

There was noticeably less edema by the second day and it was gone in less than a week. The therapist noted this on her chart and remarked that the changes were quite unusual: normally edema of this volume would take months to subside.

Her surgical incision turned white and blotchy the second day after starting *CMO*, which caused her some concern, but she continued using *CMO* anyway. The following day she noticed the incision looked better—it wasn't red or swollen.

At the time I interviewed the patient she was still in rehabilitation. Her recovery has been steady and uneventful and she seems to have regained full use of her arm. She credits *CMO* for the early rapid changes.

Extensive swelling and inflammation can be very painful as well as an obstruction to good circulation. The rapid changes she experienced could only have been due to the effects of *CMO*, because nothing else was changed during the week of her major improvements.

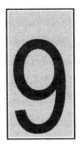

CMO AND THE BACK

A physician I know complained about long-term pain in his lower back and feet. It was difficult for him to sit very long. He often had to shove a pillow behind his back to feel any comfort at all. He had tried a back brace but found that too cumbersome. His foot pains seemed to be independent of his back. Standing on them for too long set the pain off. Once his feet were in pain they would stay sore for days unless he soaked them in warm water and massaged the soreness out. There were no foot deformities, but he had the beginnings of varicose veins on the bottoms of both feet.

He started on *CMO*, and two days later he noticed some relief. Two weeks later most of his back pains were gone. Now he rarely feels pain in his back, and if it does start up, he says, the pain goes away rather rapidly <u>without doing anything</u>. His feet still hurt a little if he stands too long, but one or two capsules of *CMO* is enough.

BACK PAINS

Back pains are the second leading symptom resulting in doctor visits for middle aged men and women. And back symptoms ranked second among complaints heard by internists and family practitioners. In my office, I would say 7 out of 10 patients complain about their back, even though that is not the reason they came to see me.

The causes for back pains are endless. If we skip disc problems and pinched nerves, the next most common problem that I see is postural strain and fascial laxity. The *fascia* is a layer of thick tissue that surrounds the body just under the skin. It helps keep things tightly in place like rolls of plastic wrap. It also separates different areas of the body into baggie-like compartments. One of its most important duties is to keep bones and soft tissues lined up in their proper positions. Looseness in the fascia can cause adjoining bones to move farther than they were intended. Pain occurs when this happens.

When tissues stretch too far they pull on the nerves. Nerves are not elastic: they don't stretch, they just hurt. The most common place for this to happen in the sacrum, the lower back. Your lower-back bone is not attached to your hip bones, it floats between them, suspended by fascia, and tightened by muscles. This is an area that can easily be strained by poor posture, overextension or flexion. Weak, unexercised muscles are a real setup for back pains.

As with foot pains, back pains often disappear with **CMO**. It all comes down to the cause: if it's related to arthritis, or some type of chronic inflammation, then there is an excellent chance **CMO** will help.

LELAND

Now I'm going to tell you the story about Leland, a retired school teacher. The surgeons have really had their way with this poor guy—seven back surgeries that have involved virtually every vertebra in his back. He even has a steel plate in his neck. He was scheduled for surgery number eight when he heard about *CMO.*

Let's look at Leland as he was just before he took *CMO.* Three fingers and the thumb on each hand were numb. He had large "nodules" surrounding most of the joints in his fingers. His doctor had labeled them bone spurs. His doctor explained that the only treatments possible were injecting the nodules with cortisone, or removing the nodules with surgery.

He was considering one or both of the options before he learned of *CMO,* because his hands were throbbing so much they kept him awake all night: He was very tired and getting depressed.

Leland's back problems were *something else!* In spite of seven surgeries he was still having excruciating pain, especially in his neck. He has been told by his doctors that large numbers of bone spurs were noticed during a 1992 lower back surgery. X rays and CAT scans exposed the spurs as well. His doctors indicated the spurs were the cause of most of his pains.

Leland's back pains have been so intense that he has had to have <u>bilateral 3-level nerve blocks</u> every month or two since the last surgery. He has also required continuous pain medications.

He started *CMO* on March 22, 1996, and stayed on 4 capsules a day for one month, then he changed to 1 daily for two weeks. At the time of this writing he has had a 50% reduction in pain, has stopped all pain medications except aspirin, and has not had to return for his nerve block. He says as time passes his pains continue to abate. He's going to wait six weeks and then restart the *CMO.*

Considering the amount of pain this man has suffered, I think a 50% reduction in pain is terrific. Especially since the agent that made the change was a nutrient, not a drug.

There is another point here to talk about: his bone spurs. The ones on his knuckles are disappearing: you can barely feel the knobs now. The throbbing in his hands has left entirely. He is sleeping through the night and feeling much better. He is planning to have another CAT scan to see if the spurs along his vertebrae are also resolving.

He is still receiving the benefits of *CMO* at this time and we won't know for several years just how much he will benefit. All we know for sure is that Leland will never stop using *CMO* when he needs it.

A PAIN FORMULA TO INCREASE *CMO*'s EFFECTIVENESS

Most people will experience 70% to 100% pain relief with *CMO*. For those who receive 70% or less relief, it's helpful to have a backup formula. I use 750 mgs of DL phenylalanine (an amino acid known to relieve pain), one or two capsules of capsaicin (hot pepper), and one or two tablets of white willow bark. It takes a few days for this formula to work so be patient.

Capsaicin works by killing small-diameter nerve fibers, the ones responsible for pain. DL phenylalanine increases the production of natural pain relieving endorphins. And white willow bark contains natural aspirin.

FIBROMYALGIA

Fibromyalgia is a generalized pain syndrome of the musculo-skeletal system, which includes tender points and diffuse areas of soreness. Usually this overlaps with chronic fatigue syndrome. Females in the 20 to 50 age range acquire it 20 times more often than men. The cause is still unknown.

Probably the worst symptom of all is the nonrestorative sleep. This may be the actual cause of fibromyalgia, according to some sleep specialists. They base this idea on studies in which volunteers were deprived of their stage IV sleep and developed the same symptoms: fatigue, pain and soreness. Another severe symptom found in fibromyalgia patients is muscular weakness. Muscle biopsies and EMG'S have been inconclusive so far.

HELGA

An 82-year-old female complained of the above symptoms. Saying she hadn't had a pain-free day in two years, she never slept more than two hours straight and seldom got more than 3 or 4 hours of actual sleep a night. She had virtually no strength left in her hands, not even enough to hold a pen for more than a minute. She was constantly tired and weak. But she couldn't sit long either: She was constantly moving from hip to hip because of the pains. Her left shoulder was in constant pain. If she moved it in a certain way the pain was so intense she would start to cry.

Helga seldom took her anti-inflammatory medicines because her stomach had become too sensitive to drugs, especially aspirin.

Apparently her stomach was able to accept *CMO* without difficulty, because on the third night she slept better than she had in years. A week later, she was still taking 2 capsules of *CMO* twice daily, and reporting no pain anywhere. Her knees even worked, she said, and she could hold a pen for the first time in a year.

She began to feel so good she decided to do some of the

projects she had neglected. She began to overdo things, an action common to those recovering from fatigue, and this caused her to have a small relapse. She cut her activities back and the recovery continued to a point where she can drive her car now without discomfort. She can sit through long sermons during church. She can work on her lawn and flower bed. And she can now sleep 6 or 7 hours a night.

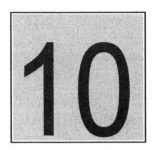

AUTOIMMUNE DISEASES

MULTIPLE SCLEROSIS

How will the folks with Multiple Sclerosis fare with **CMO**? I have treated several such patients and there has been improvement, but not as much as I had hoped for. I think it is going to take experience and inventiveness to realize **CMO's** maximum benefit to MS patients. I have combined it with other nutrients such as basic myelin protein, and my results are improving. Under no circumstance would I allow a patient to discontinue other therapies while using **CMO**. There is no need to discontinue because **CMO** is compatible with all of them.

Multiple Sclerosis *should respond* to **CMO** in a positive way because it falls under the criteria for success that I set up at the beginning of the book. It's a chronic autoimmune disease with proven depletions of essential fatty acids.

Numerous trials have indicated that Multiple Sclerosis responds to essential fatty acid therapy as well as oral tolerization therapy. MS should respond to *CMO,* too. My experience is that the symptoms of stiffness and fatigue leave almost immediately at the beginning of treatment. Patients report greater endurance and physical strength. Unfortunately these benefits seem to disappear soon after *CMO* is discontinued. It may be therefore necessary that MS patients continue the capsules indefinitely.

ADDING SPHINGOLIN (MYELIN SHEATH EXTRACT)

If you have MS, perhaps you should read Chapter 23 at the end of reading this chapter. Sphingolin is an available commercial nutrient made by a company called Ecological Research. It is authentic basic myelin protein, which is the therapeutic agent researchers have used to end MS relapse. You will need a doctor's prescription, so find an experienced physician (Call Ecological Research for Doctors) who knows how to use this and similar products. Work with him or her. Reports back to Ecological Research are that success rates with sphingolin are extremely high. Like *CMO*, sphingolin is free of side effects.

FISH OIL AND FREE RADICALS

Fish oil is a must (flax seed oil is second choice). Research has shown that autoimmune patients exhibit complex defects in the synthesis and maintenance of cellular membrane phospholipids. It is thought that these changes severely disarrange T cell lipids, causing them to become dysfunctional. You will remember the T cells, and later the B cells are the trouble makers.

Free radical activity is much greater during exacerbations of multiple sclerotic symptoms. One trigger to MS symptoms is an imbalance of fatty acids, resulting in a deficiency of EFAs. Essential acids are antioxidants in addition to being anti-inflammatories so they would obviously be helpful in the suppression of symptoms. In addition to the oils, antioxidants are called for here. Free radical activity is contributory to inflammation and its suppression is a must. SOD and glutathione (as well as other antioxidants) should be used in high doses during acute phases and in moderate doses during quiescent periods. Diet is also very important to symptom control. One must scrupulously avoid rancid fats and trans fats. Sugar is also very destructive to essential acids, and, therefore, must be restricted to smaller quantities. I suspect that the gluten grains are also involved, based upon the fact that wheat evokes high levels of serium acidity. This encourages growth of candida as well as stimulating multiple symptoms in susceptible people.

NANCY

This 52-year-old female has had MS for over 10 years. Fortunately for her, the disease's progress has been slow, with only an occasional mild flare-up. Her most difficult symptoms have been muscular weakness, fatigue, lack of endurance and depression. These symptoms seem to be with her all the time, fading then returning.

These four symptoms disappeared in less than a week after starting **CMO**. She notices she can walk twice as far on her morning hike. She never seems to be tired anymore, which allows her to keep up with the housework for the first time in years.

ROGER

Roger has been in a wheelchair for over a year. He felt like he was freezing up from all the inactivity. He had not realized until after he started the **CMO** just how little he accomplished in a day. As a businessman he needed to keep on top of things. As the sole support of his household, he needed a steady income. After taking *CMO* he noted he could move around much easier. His physical strength was amazing, he thought. His libido went from nothing to above normal. He felt this was the greatest blessing of the capsules. Unfortunately, he has not left his wheelchair because his nerves have not regenerated. We are now adding other nutrients with the hope of a future breakthrough. I'm sure *CMO* will be a contributing factor albeit not the central factor.

LUPUS

Systemic Lupus Erythematosus (SLE) is a chronic inflammatory condition characterized by arthritis, cutaneous rash, vasculitis, kidney disease and central nervous symptom dysfunction. It is an autoimmune disease. As with MS, Lupus is an involvement with a subpopulations of white blood cells, notably the T and B cells. Here again, essential oils have a proven record of retarding T cell and B cell proliferation, the cause of inflammation and tissue damage.

An article in the June 1994 issue of the Journal of Immunology reported that essential fatty acids inhibited autoimmune disease in a group of rats made ill with a disease similar to human Lupus. After the disease was induced, the rats were fed a diet containing either 10% corn oil or 10% fish oil. Symptoms of the disease occurred earlier in the corn oil group, considerably shortening their lives. Fatty acid analysis of the spleens taken from the corn-oil fed animals was found to be high in arachodonic acid and linoleic acid, a Pro-inflammatory combination.

The fish oil-fed rats had minimal symptoms and expanded survival times. Spleen cells from this group showed high levels of essential oils (n-3s), the anti-inflammatory oils.

The essential oils, fish oil in particular, not only retarded autoimmune reactions, but modulated gene expression which, additionally, slows the disease. Fish oil is able to prevent kidney damage in rat models of Lupus; it appears the antioxidant quality of the oil is the important factor here. *CMO* should be very useful here, especially when combined with fish oil and type two collagen (sold by Ecological Research, see last chapter). There are a number of studies indicating that fish oil has been immensely beneficial to Lupus. In one study, fish oil produced a prolonged remission in ten patients with Lupus. Generally speaking the amount used is around 6 gms a day (6 capsules). The average fish oil capsule contains about 1 gm of oil. Six capsules seems like a small price to pay for a partial recovery. In every study so far, there has been no reported side effects.

Turn to Chapter 23 for more information on type two collagen. This protein is a desensitizer which is harmless and inexpensive.

At least one research project mentioned the synergistic effect of taking several essential oils together. A combination of *CMO,* fish oil and flax seed oil should work well. Diet is as important here as it is in MS. One cannot eat foods that destroy essential oils (rancid fats, trans fats, etc.) and then expect much from the therapeutic nutrients—it ends up a washout.

Since insulin is pro-inflammatory, one should consider the possibility that an insulin-resistant state is hindering progress. I would certainly consider correcting the insulin resistance (hypoglycemia or diabetes) as an early step in the healing process. Look in the section on vanadyl sulfate for a method of doing this.

NOTE

Both sphingolin and collagen type 2 can be obtained from Ecological Formulas, 1061-B, Shary Circle, Concord, California 94518. 800-888-4585.

JERRY

In his mid 50s, Jerry was diagnosed with Lupus ten years before. His cheeks are always rosy red because of his circulation. His joints are painful, as are his muscles. He doesn't sleep well, so that contributes to his excessive fatigue. He has difficulty controlling his bladder and his occasional pains in the location of his kidneys.

His disease has been progressing in spite of medications. He came to see me, wondering if a nutritional approach might help. I put him on *CMO*, type two collagen, manganese, proline and gave him vitamin injections. I also put him on a sleep medication, which I later changed to melatonin. His aches and pains left within several weeks. His energy came up rapidly and he felt more positive about his future. His muscles are much stronger so he has good bladder control again. We'll take each day as it comes from now on, working to keep him in remission, reacting to what ever happens: As for now—so far, so good.

DIABETES

Diabetes is considered by many doctors to be a smoldering inflammation, an autoimmune disease. There may be different causes for diabetes, one being an autoimmune reaction. If so, it would increase the likelihood of your responding to **CMO.**

As if it weren't enough that diabetics suffer a deficiency of essential oils, the disease spins off a number of other diseases that also result in deficits of EFAs.

Diabetics, both animal and humans, have been found to have fewer EFAs. Not only is heart disease more prevalent in deficient subjects, but so is hypertension. The same mechanisms are involved here, whether it's the coronary artery, the iliac arteries, or the carotid arteries. Once the arterial wall is damaged from free radicals, the plaguing starts in earnest. Not only does plaguing contribute to hypertension, but the loss of the arterial relaxing factor, nitric oxide, results from high levels of free radical activity.

Diabetics often have dyslipidemia. Low density lipoproteins (LPLs) are higher in their blood, thus diabetics have a greater than normal likelihood of developing atherosclerosis and coronary heart disease. Apparently the LPLs are able to invade the diabetic's artery walls. Once in, they are easily oxidized by the high levels of free radicals so frequently found in diabetics.

It is well known that diabetics will develop atherosclerosis at a younger age. The explanation may be related to the 40% increase over normal in LPLs seen in the serium of diabetics.

The brains of diabetic rats exhibit a decreased capacity for glucose oxidation and an increased capacity for fatty acid oxidation. Diabetics who are poorly controlled could be potentially in danger of serious alterations of brain metabolism. This altered brain chemistry can produce an encephalopathy.

The eye, as part of the brain, is just as susceptible to this degeneration. Maculopathy is common to diabetics: half of the blindness in this country is due to poorly controlled diabetes.

Nerves seem to degenerate in the diabetic over time. The sciatic nerve, for example, is a common location for diabetic neuropathy. In one study, blood flow to the sciatic nerve of diabetics was reduced by 47%. Not only are the nerves damaged directly, the circulation to the nerves is restricted. This interference to leg circulation due to complications of diabetes is behind half of the leg amputations in this country. Obesity probably adds to this problem because it is one of those diseases intimately connected to insulin imbalance.

Regarding obesity, linoleic acid, an EFA, has been found to be deficient in the fat cells of diabetics. Low levels of this oil in the fat cells are indirectly related to sudden cardiac deaths. This statistic was taken from 84 men between ages 25 to 64 who suddenly died of a heart attack within 24 hours of cardiac symptoms. None of these men had a prior history of heart disease or were medically treated for hyperlipidemia. Their blood lipids were compared to 292 healthy men. There was a 95% correlation between the levels of EFAs in the fat cells of men who suddenly died and those who did not.

VITAMIN E HELPS

Daily administration of Vitamin E to diabetics caused a reduction in plasma glucose, triglycerides, free fatty acids, total cholesterol, LPLs and apoprotein B. Vitamin E did not help the beta cells in the pancreas make more insulin though.

A study in the Annals of the New York Academy of Sciences, June 1993, showed that fish oil provided the very same laboratory improvements as vitamin E to all of the tests listed above. In both studies, glucose levels improved.

Fish oil has additional benefits to the diabetic by acting on insulin receptors. It apparently improves the effects of insulin around the body while decreasing its effects in the liver where insulin needs to be less active. Fish oil makes insulin more powerful to the tissues, thus reducing the need for so much insulin.

In general, Eskimos who still live as their ancestors did, rarely develop diabetes or arteriosclerosis. This, in spite of the fact that as much as 80% of their food is oil. Fish oil in enormous quantities seems to retard these two degenerative diseases.

Another benefit of fish oil is that it is an anticoagulant. In a study in the Journal Arteriosclerosis and Thrombosis, August 1993, 15,000 people were sampled as to diets to determine whether dietary fatty acid intake influenced blood levels of coagulation proteins. The results indicate that EFAs from fish oil thin the blood by modifying the blood levels of the coagulation factors.

I add vanadyl sulfate when I use *CMO* on diabetics because this metal ion can greatly improve the effects of insulin. And it works within as little as three weeks. When diabetic rats were given intra-abdominal injections of vanadyl sulfate, their serum glucose levels dropped to normal in two days. This is probably because vanadyl sulfate acts in some ways like a substitute insulin without all of the negative qualities of insulin.

RENA

I accepted this young insulin dependent diabetic for nutritional therapy, with some reservations. Normally this type of diabetic is unresponsive to nutritional intervention. My experience with her treatment has changed my mind.

I should start the story by commenting on her extraordinary cooperation and dedication to her health improvement. This patient was willing to test her blood sugar frequently and keep excellent records. If she had not done this our efforts would have failed.

She took *CMO* along with other nutrients, and then rearranged the types and dosages as we went along. Very soon I added vanadyl sulfate, taurine, chromium, zinc, vitamin E, EFAs and various supporting nutrients.

She came in with a blood sugar wildly out of control. Changing the type of insulin, the amount or time of day taken, did not control the blood sugar. The blood sugar fluctuated radically from 180 to well over 300. As we began treatment blood sugars stayed in the 300's, a worrisome turn. At this early stage she could have quit panic and I wouldn't have blamed her.

But Rena had true grit and she stayed in the battle. We, together, adjusted doses, nutritional mixes, diet, insulin and everything else we could think of.

After, what seemed like forever, the blood sugar averaged started down. Whew!! It kept going down—and down—and down. She lowered her insulin but could not do without it.

The blood sugar began to stabilize, and desist from it's erratic peaks and valleys. It leveled off at 110, rising modestly after eating.

I will explore the subject of vanadyl and insulin more in Chapter 21. As for now, let me just say that *CMO* has its benefit to the diabetic, but it should be accompanied by other synergistic nutrients for the full benefit.

SOURCES

SOD as SOD Complex is available from GERO VITA at 800-694-8366.

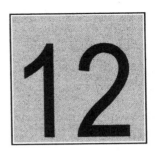

HYPERTENSION

Of all the diseases I have ever treated, I think hypertension has been the hardest disease to overcome. Drugs work, of course, but I'm speaking of the use of nutrients against high blood pressure.

What about magnesium? I've been told, as have many of you, that the best nutrient for hypertension is magnesium. To tell you the truth, I have never seen it work for hypertension. If it hasn't worked for you either, join the crowd. I can also add that I have never interviewed a patient who has had success with magnesium under another doctor's direction either. You may read a great deal about magnesium in popular literature, but as far as I'm concerned, magnesium is not a treatment for hypertension.

I'd like to add that garlic oil, often touted as a cure for hypertension, has also been a complete flop.

Up until recently I hadn't found much else that worked either. That's why I became so excited when I heard about **CMO**. My excitement over **CMO** stirred me into a review of nutrients and hypertension where I found an abundance of material on the EFAs. That really got my hopes up. I've helped many more people with hypertension since then.

During my library research on hypertension I found over a hundred studies indicating that EFAs, and fish oil in particular, act to lower blood pressure.

One of the earlier studies was a comparison between a mackerel diet and a herring diet for hypertension. 15 men agreed to adhere to one or the other diet for 2 weeks. The herring diet produced a modest lowering of blood lipids and blood pressure. The mackerel diet brought the blood pressure and the blood lipids down significantly. The conclusion was that the type of fish or fish oil was important.

DRUGS AND HYPERTENSION

Many would say, why bother? After all, we have perfectly good drugs for hypertension, so why poke around for something else. Take a moment and think: you already know the answer.

New drugs for hypertension always look good at the beginning. Most side effects are tolerable and they seem to work. But things change after a while. Even though these drugs control blood pressure, they don't stop the steady progression of the disease. Hypertensive medications artificially lower blood pressure, ignoring the fundamental underlying cause.

Hypertension continues, and after a while the patient is told he will have to take **more medicine**, then **change to a stronger medicine**, **then add a second medicine**, **then add a third medicine**, and so on. The disease continues to worsen in spite of the drugs. NOW. Do you really believe drugs are the final answer to this problem?

Another problem with drugs: After years of usage, doctors are seeing long-term organ damage. Some of these drugs cause premature heart failure, kidney disease, or liver damage.

Some doctors would argue that high blood pressure would have done patients in earlier anyway, the drugs actually extended their life. This argument ignores the fact that there were other options to consider in the beginning. Nutritional approaches to hypertension treat the cause not the symptom, while not adding health risks.

NUTRITIONAL FACTORS IN HYPERTENSION

There is a controversy regarding the type of essential oil that works best with hypertension. One group favors fish oil while another says that evening primrose oil is the best. Of course, one could easily suspend the argument by trying one of the oils, and if it didn't work, try the other. EFAs do not have side effects, generally, so what would be the risk?

Fish oil has another effect on blood pressure. It reduces the response in the arterial wall to adrenaline. Adrenaline causes the artery to constrict, and the failure of the relaxing response keeps it semipermanently tight.

Another nutrient that adds to the hypertensive effect of fish oil is vitamin E. It is known to normalize lipid peroxidation and stabilize the enzymes actively involved in the antioxidant balance.

If the diet is low in potassium, then the blood pressure is more likely to be high. Potassium and magnesium seem to balance sodium. So if sodium is high and the other two are low the blood pressure is under pressure to rise.

The dietary restriction of sodium and the addition of EFAs seems to make the response to fish oil decidedly stronger. Another interesting fact is that none of these nutrients lower normal blood pressures. Yes, it's been tested, but it failed. Those with normal blood pressures should have <u>no</u> fear of developing low blood pressure.

I consider low blood pressure to be as dangerous as hypertension. Low blood pressure is a first symptom of an unstable balance of the system. As the balance worsens the low pressures will flip into high pressures. This is not new information, it's been documented for years, and ignored by doctors who find low blood pressures and tell the patients "you are going to live forever with a blood pressure like this".

While the fish oil is lowering blood pressure it is also lowering cholesterol and thinning the blood. Not a bad idea if one has coronary risk factors as well. Another positive is that cardiac hypertrophy (enlarged heart), has been reduced while using fish oil for hypertension. This could be expected, of course, but it's always nice to see it actually happen.

Fish oil can even be combined with a drug to enhance the value of both. When fish oil was combined with nifedipine it produced a lower blood pressure than either singularly.

RELAXING FACTORS

Some individuals have the type of blood pressure that shoots up during stress. We've all heard of the person who goes to his doctor and his blood pressure spikes from the stress of the examination. At home, this same individual may check himself on a home monitoring device and find a normal blood pressure (assuming his medications are working). Mistakenly, doctors assume this type of elevation is so temporary that it can be ignored.

But we shouldn't ignore it because this individual is demonstrating an additional inability to relax arteries. There is every reason to believe that blood pressure which rises under the stress of a doctor visit will probably rise under many stressful circumstances. But it won't be measured, so this individual will not know that it's happening.

This condition occurs as a failure of the relaxing factor in the artery wall. It's a malfunction in the endothelial (inner surface of the artery) lining. Something is seriously wrong with the artery. Why wait till it drifts further off balance? Why not take care of it BEFORE it becomes a full blown disaster?

The major relaxing factor in most arterial walls is a substance called nitric oxide. It, in itself, is a free radical and capable of damaging tissue. Most of the time, though, it does more good than harm. One of the substances that seems to activate its relaxing qualities are the EFAs. This is because the EFAs have antioxidant effects. The most powerful antioxidant known to enhance the relaxing effects of nitric oxide is SOD, superoxide dismutase, and its sister, glutathione. **When we use large doses of these two antioxidants, we see the blood pressure dropping toward normal**, but one has to be patient, as it doesn't happen overnight. I'll tell you more about it at the end of the chapter.

ECLAMPSIA

All pregnant females who develop hypertension should be taking magnesium (the one time when it does reverse hypertension), fish oil and evening primrose oil. These three nutrients are capable of eliminating eclampsia. You would think in this day and age everybody would have heard about this formula, but they haven't.

VEINS

When we talk about hypertension the arteries are the focus of attention. We never talk about the veins, and yet, the blood must return to the heart somehow. We assume the veins are big, wide open pipes. Not so, studies have shown that hypertension and obesity, together, seriously compromise the veins. These diseases do it by reducing venous distensibility, preventing expansion of the walls. The functional factors behind this are just as important as the structural factors.

Venous blood is not healthy. It carries metabolic waste, unlike the nourishing factors found in arterial blood. Veins are actually a sewer system, and any time they are sledged up or slowed they will back up everything behind them, leaving the tissues to wallow in their own garbage. In one sense, you can think of arteries as faucets and veins as drains—which can back up.

It is just as important for the veins to be free-flowing as the arteries. Arteries get the groceries to the door, but it is the veins that keep the place sanitary. And you know, unsanitary conditions lead to disease.

When the arteries are affected by a disease, so are the veins, although it won't be as noticeable.

INSULIN RESISTANCE

Another factor that is associated closely with hypertension is insulin resistance. Whenever you have insulin resistance you have high levels of insulin. Insulin has a number of effects, including its lesser known pro-inflammatory quality, which contributes to arteriosclerosis and failing arterial wall relaxing factors.

CONCLUDING REMARKS

One of the most common questions asked is whether the endothelial dysfunction in hypertensives is reversible. The answer is—No!—if you are suggesting drugs as the mechanism of change. Drugs have not been proven to restore endothelial function. There is some proof, however, that chronic lipid-lowering therapy is effective in restoring endothelial function both in the coronary and peripheral circulation. It takes years to do it though.

Drugs never do it.

If you have hypertension don't be afraid to take **CMO**. There have been no reports of it increasing blood pressure. To the contrary, there are a number of reports of blood pressure decreasing. **CMO**, as far as we know, has not interacted with blood pressure medicines.

Can **CMO** improve your high blood pressure? It might, especially if you combine it with other nutrients such as EFAs, SOD, glutathione and coenzyme Q 10 (see Chapter 22).

OSCAR

A Nebraska farmer was having difficulty with impotency as a result of 6 years on hypertensive medications. His average BP was 165/100 and it wasn't well-controlled with the medications. In addition to his family physician, the patient saw a chiropractor and was placed on a diet with the expectation it might improve his cholesterol and his blood pressure.

He was given **CMO** by his chiropractor because he complained of daily stiffness and aching in both knees. Neither doctor nor patient suspected **CMO** would affect the blood pressure. 5 weeks later the patient's knees were, according to him, "tremendously improved". There was some stiffness but the pain was entirely gone. As a matter of course his blood pressure was checked during the office visit and found to be 132/86. He was told by the chiropractor to see his family physician about reducing the medication. He told the doctor he hadn't taken his blood pressure medications in over 2 weeks.

CAL

Cal had been on two different blood pressure medications for years, but had seen his pressure steadily rise just the same. When we first met, his systolic blood pressure (the top one) was bobbing from 150 to over 200, and the diastolic was ranging 100 to 115.

His family physician was constantly changing the dose of each medicine and had warned him a third medication was next. I placed him on **CMO**, coenzyme Q 10, taurine, fish oil and minerals.

It took months, and a lot of patience, but the pressures gradually dropped despite our eliminating one of his medicines. But still his blood pressure would spike during stress.

The nutrient that eventually controlled the spiking was SOD (see the list of resources in the last chapter). <u>SOD increases the amount of relaxing factors in arterial walls</u>. For the first time in 20 years this patient's systolic blood pressure averaged 130 to 140, with the diastolic at 70. Spiking was less frequent and popped up to about 150.

Cal is still on a half a blood pressure pill as we continue to work the formula.

CMO made a difference along with all of the other nutrients. In the beginning it was a combination of factors that made his blood pressure rise abnormally, and in the end it was a combination of factors that made it normal.

SOURCES

SOD as SOD Complex is available from GERO VITA at 800-694-8366.

13

CMO AND
THE CHRONIC GUT

PRESCRIPTION MEDICATIONS

This is probably as good a place as any to talk about prescription medicines. If you are on medications from your doctor for any disease, don't stop taking them. Continue your medications *AND* take **CMO** at the same time. When your symptoms disappear, ask your doctor to lower or discontinue your medicines.

Experience has shown that medications do not undermine the benefits of **CMO** and vice versa. Therefore, use them both simultaneously. <u>It is important that you not discontinue valuable treatments in order to experiment with a nutrient for which the outcome is not 100% assured</u>. While there is an excellent chance it will work, there is no guarantee. It's much safer if you use **CMO** and your medicine at the same time.

I have talked to many of the doctors who use **CMO** therapy and all of them admit they have used it for many ailments other than arthritis. In fact, I think the consensus of opinion is that it should be tried on all diseases including mental illnesses, and this includes schizophrenia. There are no tests to say who will respond and who will not, so no one knows for sure whether it will work until they try it.

Pay attention, use proper care, and no harm should come from trying it.

CMO AND GASTROINTESTINAL DISEASES

HERBERT

Herbert is a 41-year-old uptight lawyer with a wife, no kids and Crohn's disease. He has been on a very restrictive diet to alleviate frequent abdominal pains, tons of gas, an occasional fever and rectal bleeding. In fact, he's rushed himself to the hospital twice with rectal bleeding.

After a barium enema showed a narrow gut, Herbert was placed on aspirins and oral steroids, then later he was placed on azatheoprine. Stress seems to kick up the symptoms and, of course, he has lots of that. He's been told he'll have to learn to live with his disease, which is depressing for him to hear.

Crohn's, a disease of unknown causes, is an inflammation of the small and large intestine. It may be triggered by stress but it's probably a genetic disease. Spontaneous regressions are few and far between. And there is no known medical cure, although the symptoms can be treated successfully.

Herbert took the *CMO* treatment and improved by 80% in six weeks, then he decided to repeat, seeking further improvement; 90% of the time he is free of symptoms, but he is still planning another round of *CMO* when he can. His doctor requested another barium study, but Herbert has declined, feeling that he knows he's better and doesn't have to prove it to the doctor.

Herbert's two very minor flare-ups during the first 6 months following the original treatment were quickly eliminated by a few capsules of *CMO*. He accepts the fact that he is not completely cured, but his symptoms are pretty much controlled and he feels like a new man.

Although maybe not the result of the *CMO,* his anxieties are lower too, as are his reactions to stress. I have seen *CMO* reduce anxiety and depression in others, and I tend to think some of the emotional improvements may have been due to *CMO*. I used other nutrients along with the *CMO,* which I will describe in the last case of this chapter.

ESSENTIAL FATTY ACIDS AND BOWEL DISEASE

Essential fatty acids are known to improve the symptoms of Crohn's, as well as all of the other inflammatory bowel diseases. To prove my point—that essential oils are restorative to inflammations of the gut—let's look at 6 examples, pulled from a large file of research papers.

1. A November 1995 issue of the Journal of Gastroenterology ran an article which said that when there was more EFAs in the diet there was reduced damage to the colon. What EFAs actually do, it said, was to suppress leukotriene B4, which is an inflammatory eicosanoid. In other words, EFAs suppress the chemicals that cause the burning and soreness.

2. A January 1996 article that appeared in the Journal of Metabolism: Clinical and Experimental stated that patients with chronic intestinal disorders have biochemical evidence of essential fatty acid deficiencies and elevated arachidonic acid, (AAs: arachidonic acid

is behind the inflammatory eicosanoid hormones), more on this in Chapter 24. Mono-unsaturated fatty acids (MUFAs) were also high in chronic inflammatory gut diseases. The mono's (MUFAs) weakly encourage inflammation, too.

Once again we see imbalances in the thinning and hardening oils. It's the same no matter where the inflammation is located: it just happens to be in the gut in this case. The imbalance is such that there is a deficiency of firefighters (EFAs), and a glut of firestarters (AAs and MUFAs)

3. In January 1993, an article in Gut stated that abnormal plasma unsaturated fatty acids have been reported in active irritable bowel syndrome (IBD). The authors thought that there was probably a primary deficiency of EFAs in patients with IBD.

4. In the Annals of Internal Medicine, September 92 issue, it was noted that a 4-month diet supplemented with fish oil in patients with inflammatory bowel disease resulted in reductions in symptoms of ulcerative colitis.

5. Other oils work too. Alimentary Pharmacology and Therapeutics, April 1993, said that evening primrose oil seemed to change some of the symptoms of colitis and was beneficial as a treatment.

6. More dramatically, the European Journal of Clinical Investigation in November 1993 reported that EFAs were given intravenously to a 36-year-old female with ulcerative colitis and severe steroid side effects. 200 ml of fish oil, a derived lipid emulsion, was infused for 9 days.

Disease activity in the colon declined rapidly and the patient was transferred to 16 fish oil capsules daily for two months afterwards. When the fish oil was stopped, the severe symptoms of colitis rapidly recurred.

The same IV treatments were repeated for 29 more days, during which her symptoms completely disappeared and did not return, as far as the researchers could tell, by the time of publication.

I have a large collection of similar references, all indicating that chronic bowel disease is associated with a disturbance in essential oils.

GASTROINTESTINAL INFLAMMATIONS AND *CMO*

You can see from this small sampling that essential fatty acids are helpful to those with inflammations along the GI tract. *CMO* is very beneficial to this group of bowel diseases because it is so effective against chronic inflammation.

Let me end the subject of gastrointestinal diseases with two more examples.

NANCY

Nancy is a 50-year-old business woman who was irritable, and had trouble staying on a diet. The diet she was struggling with relieved her symptoms of ulcerative colitis when she followed it. She was almost addicted to aspirin enemas, her only reliable form of relief.

When a barium enema showed cobblestoning in the gut, her internist put her on cortisone. She would get colicky and feverish every so often, especially when she went to a business lunch and gobbled down the wrong things.

CMO gave her fair relief, but she was disappointed and hypercritical. We repeated the entire treatment schedule a month later, with better success the second time. So far she is doing well. One change that others most appreciate is her kinder personality. She wasn't really as mean and spiteful as she acted, she just felt bad most of the time.

One precaution: If you are planning to use *CMO* for ulcers, please be careful. Take care to eat food with the capsules or your ulcer will flare up instantly.

ESSE

This 44-year-old woman has been struggling with Crohn's for 6 years. She uses medications frequently, because the smallest dietary misstep flares up the symptoms. She has cramping, diarrhea, gas, soreness and all the complaints of a woman in distress. This disease has affected her work, her homelife and her self-esteem. She doesn't blame herself for having the disease, but she is depressed over its unsettling influence on her life.

I started her on *CMO* alone and it made an immediate difference. Next I added fish oil and aloe vera, vitamin A and injections of B vitamins. Each item helped make a little more improvement.

I finally added peppermint oil and hydrochloric acid and pepsin. She has been symptom-free since we started, for the most part. Dietary indiscretions have created some soreness, although nothing like she had previously experienced.

Basically, we must keep her symptom-free for a year or two until her body accepts the new balance that doesn't include inflammation. Repairing a chronically disturbed area is a long process, but it breaks up the symptom-drug-symptom-drug roller coaster ride.

Doctors are clear on disease and on treatment drugs. What they are unclear on is that it is necessary to rebalance the disturbed system in order to cure the disease. This process requires the patient to artificially maintain a new balance for a considerable length of time until the body **accepts** this new and better balance.

FOOD ALLERGIES AND THE CHRONIC GUT

If I were you I would not use *CMO* on any gut problem until you have determined your food allergies. This simple procedure should be done first because *CMO* does not correct food allergies, instead it reduces swelling and inflammation. Reactive foods will bring all these problems back again quickly.

The most common irritant to the bowel is **WHEAT!** All grains can irritate the gut, but wheat is the worst. Rye or rice may seem safer than wheat, don't count on it. I have seen a number of individuals react adversely to rice. Soy beans, the darling of the vegetarians, is always suspect.

The next most common irritant to the gut is sugar, but then you've probably already suspected that. Fruit sugars will occasionally cause the same intense reactions.

Then comes dairy. Dairy includes anything that has even the smallest trace of milk in it. Soups may contain milk solids for example. **Read your labels!**

TESTING FOR FOOD ALLERGIES

Let's test all three of these suspicious foods at the same time. Bravely give them up for a full week (not a single bite mind you, even ONE exposure will ruin the test). Your gut symptoms should have improved during this week. If they weren't then it is less likely you are food sensitive.

On day one of the following week, add back into your diet as much wheat and grains as you can eat. Continue to read labels and avoid milk products or items with sugar (including chocolate).

If you are wheat or grain intolerant then you are going to have one miserable day. You will probably be bursting with gas which may cause cramping. You may also develop diarrhea, fatigue, moodiness, headaches and other symptoms. To abort the misery stop the grains and take baking soda in water. An Alka-Seltzer may be of great help at this time. Now you have learned a food group which keeps your gut chronically inflamed.

The next day, drink and overeat as much dairy as you can. Avoid grains and sugar. If dairy is a problem you will have the same reaction as you did to grains. If you react then treat it the same as I described with wheat.

Use sugar on the third day repeating the same process.

If you really do have a food intolerance you are now well aware of it, in fact you might be quite sick right now. I guess I don't have to tell you what to avoid in the future.

You are probably asking yourself how can you desensitize to these foods? It can be done, but that, I'm afraid is the subject for another book. But now at least, you know that edibles are not always food friendly.

DO NOT CONFUSE YOURSELF

CMO is not useful for food allergies, although it is terrific for gut inflammations. You need to clarify your food sensitivities and withdraw from them *before* you use *CMO* for any type of inflamed gut. If you continue to eat the offending foods you will probably and falsely conclude that *CMO* didn't work.

OTHER NUTRITIONAL AIDS

Colitis and similar gut conditions have responded to *medium chain fatty acids*. These non-fattening oils come in a quart container like flax oil and are known to soothe the gut wall. They can be mixed in foods, taken straight, or used for cooking. Numerous studies have connected them to gut healing. Call Life Extension Products at 800-543-3873 for a supply.

Vitamin A strengthens the lining of all body cavities, including the small and large bowel, and so protects tissues.

There is some evidence that Crohn's patients respond to bovine cartilage (available in most health food stores). To this I would add Acidophyllus and Bifidus.

Last but not least is the fabulously effective dynamic duo, hydrochloric/pepsin tablets and peppermint oil capsules. When this kicks in (along with *CMO*) it's all over for your disease.

14

SKIN DISEASES

Perhaps I should start this section by telling you about a young lady who had an undiagnosed, eczema-appearing rash on the back of both hands. I say undiagnosed because every dermatologist who examined the rash offered a different opinion. The only thing they agreed on was that it wasn't eczema.

It looked like eczema and itched like eczema, but it wasn't eczema. The ghastly sight of it humiliated the patient so much she refused to shake hands at an introduction, making some weak excuse. She wore long blousy sleeves and slipped her hands up into her sleeves if she was around someone.

She would not reach for items in stores if anyone was near. The patient wore gloves when she was forced to, but they made her hands sweat and the rash worse. Sunlight made the hands burn and ache, so driving anywhere around town was a painful task.

From what I've said you've probably guessed that all of the medicines, salves, creams, powders, lotions and chemicals failed to make it better. Cortisone made the rash sting and all the rest of the medicines aggravated the itch and inflamed it.

Doctors were so frustrated with her they suggested skin grafts. They did everything they could to palm her off on someone else.

She had a sad resignation in her eyes on her first visit, hoping for help but doubting it would come. I had just gotten a new supply of *CMO* capsules and cream, so it was going to be a new therapy for her. To tell you the truth I didn't have much hope either, but why not try. I didn't believe *CMO* would harm her. If her rash flared up it would be no worse than what she'd experienced with the prescription medicines.

She started the capsules and worked the *CMO* cream into the rash twice a day. My first relief came after several days when she said the rash had not gotten worse. My second relief came two weeks later when she reported some signs of improvement. At the end of 4 weeks the rash was gone. Unfortunately, the skin had been so damaged it was blotchy and thin.

Four weeks after she stopped the cream and capsules, the rash started to reappear. She restarted the routine and it cleared again. It's too early to know how long she will have to be on the *CMO* treatment, yet it IS keeping an intolerable pre-cancerous disease under control. I told her to continue seeking a more accurate diagnosis and treatment. *CMO* would be there for her if she needed it.

To date, she hasn't found anything better.

WHAT TYPES OF SKIN DISEASES RESPOND TO *CMO*?

There are three that I know of, others may be discovered later. Those diseases are Eczema, Psoriasis and some cases of Atopic dermatitis.

WHY SHOULD SKIN DISEASES RESPOND TO *CMO*?

We are back to square one again—the answer is the essential fatty acid connection. Yes, it's true. These three diseases are known to improve on the EFAs.

FISH OIL

6 grams of fish oil were given daily, in one study, to 145 patients with diagnosed atopic dermatitis, an average 30% improvement ensued after 4 months. Where fish oil works, so does *CMO*, according to my thinking.

In a comparison study, fish oil against liquid paraffin under occlusive dressing; fish oil easily won. The disease being treated was psoriasis, and the symptoms were erythema (redness), scaling, plaque thickness and itching. Fish oil was considerably better than the paraffin.

A theoretical model for psoriasis appeared in Medical Hypotheses, May 1992. The author proposed that essential fatty acid metabolism played a crucial role both in the pathogenesis and treatment of psoriasis. Patients with psoriasis are known to have an increased generation of free radicals, which is one of the causes for the depletion of the EFAs.

PSORIASIS

One of the most useful techniques against patches of psoriasis that cannot be hidden by clothes is to apply *CMO* cream on top of the patch and cover it with waterproof tape. If you add a little over the counter cortisone it works even better. Don't disturb it for one to three weeks. Do not freshen it up every few days, just leave it alone. Try it on one small area to begin with and if it clears the patch use it on a large area. Fifty to sixty percent will probably have complete skin clearing.

Occluding the lesion with tape decreases excessive skin growth (the cause of psoriasis). It also super-hydrates the area making it clear.

You can use the oral form of *CMO* at the same time.

There is another excellent helpmate to *CMO* and that is desiccated bovine thymus which is available at most health food stores. I have my patients take quite a few tablets each day. Recently a Russian study had great success in treating psoriasis using the injectable form of thymus.

The finding from the study showed those who were successful (79%) needed only 4 to 5 follow-up injections each year to retard relapses. Thymus injections can be obtained from alternative care physicians. Apothecure, a Texas based pharmacy (800-969-6601), has a list of physicians who use this treatment. The phone for *CMO* is 800-249-7816.

Psoriasis affects one percent of the population and is caused by excessive proliferation of skin cells—cause unknown.

Normal skin cells, are born in the deepest levels of the skin, and migrate to the surface in 28 to 44 days. Skin cells migration takes only 4 days in the psoritic. You can see mounds of thick epidermal layers form, which quickly dry out and fracture off as thick silvery scales resembling mica.

ECZEMA

Eczema responds slowly to *CMO* cream—just rub it in 2 or 3 times a day, it takes about a month to really work, but you'll probably notice some early changes within two weeks.

Eczema has been found to be caused by a defect in the function of the enzyme delta-6-desaturase. This enzyme is responsible for the conversion of linoleic acid to gamma linolenic acid. Several plants, including evening primrose, are known to be rich in gamma linolenic acid.

It's possible that people prone to developing atopic eczema can be rescued by using gamma linolenic acid. A number of trials have confirmed marked improvement in atopic eczema using gamma linolenic acid. Patients showed less inflammation, dryness, scaling and overall severity compared to controls.

ATOPIC DERMATITIS

The best technique for treating Atopic Dermatitis (which is caused by a disturbance in the sweating mechanism) is to take three one minute showers a day to remove all sweat. Make sure you don't allow any soap to touch the lesions, and especially not to remain on them. Towel off and apply a mixture of over the counter cortisone cream with *CMO* cream. Improvements should start right away.

15

LUNG DISEASES

EMPHYSEMA

Both emphysema and bronchitis respond to **CMO**.

Emphysema is more commonly called chronic obstructive pulmonary disease, or COPD, nowadays. Symptoms of this disease are a permanent reduction in forced expiration, reduced vital capacity, dyspnea and wheezing. Emphysema is a permanent enlargement of the air sacs in the lungs with fibrosis and wall thickening.

Chronic bronchitis is defined as cough and hypersecretion of mucus for at least 3 months of each year.

Asthma is not the main cause for emphysema because it is only a temporary obstruction. 15,000,000 people have COPD and smoking is the main cause. Emphysema accounts for 17,000,000 office visits per year, it's ranked 5th as a cause of death. Other contributors to this disease are inorganic dusts, coal, cement, grain dusts, and acid fumes.

The underlying pathology is a chronic inflammation which

results from chronic irritation (cigarette smoke). The cardinal symptoms of emphysema are progressive dyspnea, cough, phlegm and wheezing.

A 1994 study in the New England Journal of Medicine showed that fish oil can interfere with lung inflammation and so is of benefit to those with COPD. 8,960 people were questioned, and an estimate of fatty acid intake was determined by a dietary questionnaire. The presence of COPD was assessed from three symptoms listed on the test: Symptoms of chronic bronchitis, physician-diagnosed emphysema and spirometrically-detected COPD. The conclusion was that smoking causes emphysema, but diets with high levels of essential fatty acids interfere with the development of emphysema in smokers.

How do you know whether your emphysema is severe or not? Your doctor will tell you what your forced expiratory volume is. Use this scale: 70% mild, 60% mild, 50% moderately severe, 35% very severe. Serious obstruction in the lungs often leads to right ventricular heart failure. Death comes more often from the damage it does to the heart than to lack of oxygenation.

SO WHAT DO WE KNOW?

Emphysema responds to fish oil in a very positive way and it responds in the same way to *CMO*, only faster.

KATE

A middle aged woman with chronic emphysema took *CMO* primarily to alleviate osteoarthritis of her neck and upper back. She had worked for years at a job that required her head to be forward over a table and bent down.

An electronic spirometer was used to check her lungs. There was a decrease in her vital capacity and her forced expiration. 10 days after starting *CMO* she was reexamined using the spirometer again. Her vital capacity had increased by 7% and her force exhalation was normal. She reported a big change in her ability to breathe.

ADDITIONAL NUTRIENTS FOR EMPHYSEMA

If I were treating a patient for Pulmonary Fibrosis I would start with *CMO*, then add vitamin E 1200 units a day, taurine 1500 mgs a day, niacin (long acting) 1000 mgs a day and superoxide dismutase from GETO VITA. There is substantial research evidence that the latter four elements have retarded the growth of pulmonary fibrosis. Vitamin E, in particular, has been effective in softening a number of types of fibrosis.

CAUTION

There are a number of anecdotal reports of asthma improving on *CMO*. At this time I am not advising its use in asthma, because of side effects related to allergies. I have seen asthmatics worsen on *CMO*, but I think the problem was due to dosage uncertainties. Asthmatics may require tiny doses at the start, gradually building to higher doses near the end of treatment.

Asthma turns out to be the one exception to the fish oil connection. Fish oil does, over long months, change the degree of symptoms in asthmatics.

There are a number of research trials that indicate fish oil is excellent for asthmatics. Unfortunately, this is not a defined area yet.

The unusual response to *CMO*, in asthmatics, may have to do with special receptors in the tracheal/bronchial tree called adenosine receptors. Adenosine receptors help suppress inflammation—except they make the inflammation worse in the respiratory system of the asthmatic. More of this in Chapter 24.

16

AGING

Twenty-five years from now three quarters of a million Americans will be over a hundred years old. This is not good news if another statistic doesn't change: Half of those over 85, according to the records, are dependent upon others for care. Living longer doesn't mean beans if you can't be fully functional and self-sufficient.

Life extension must include the extension of mental and physical faculties. System after system slips off balance and begins to deteriorate. We focus our attention too much on acute diseases because we know how quickly a heart attack can do us in. But we must not forget that Alzheimers and senility are diseases that isolate us and destroy our personalities as well as our vitality in life, and they are lurking around out there just waiting for their chance.

The sensory system is a good example of what I'm saying. When hearing declines, for example, a lot more is lost than the ability to communicate. Endless studies have indicated that sound is tied to frontal brain wave speed. Without constant stimulation frontal brain wave speeds slow, and as they slow, so does thinking. Called attention deficit disorder (ADD), it can accelerate mental deterioration. Children with ADD respond by becoming perennial dreamers, uninvolved with their surroundings, or they become hyperactive. Elderly people often become paranoid, depressed or withdrawn due to ADD.

As of now, 35 million Americans are over the age of 65, but in another quarter century they will exceed 70 million. Most of those people are going to live another 30 or 35 years: 3/4 of a million of them will already be over the age of 100. Pretty soon people will be so age-resistant you won't be able to kill them with a stick.

None of these people will find happiness in a debilitating disease that renders them dependent. Heart disease, hypertension, arthritis and hearing problems now represent 60% of all diseases of aging.

DOES CETYL MYRISTOLEATE REVERSE AGING?

YES!

The answer is yes, if, by that we mean *CMO* helps the diseases which cause premature aging. I think *CMO* is normally found in the human body (perhaps in a slightly different form than is found in the rat) and it depletes with age exactly as many other nutrients do, especially the antioxidants. If supplemental antioxidants can slow aging and diseases that accelerate aging, then so can *CMO*. I think periodic use of *CMO* will cause bodily tissues to remain younger and thus retard aging. If we have more of it then we will continue to be youthful.

This is of course gross speculation but then the conclusions that I draw are reasonable when you see the surprising changes brought by *CMO*.

The most common disease of aging has to do with the inner lining of our circulatory system: atherosclerosis.

ATHEROGENICITY

High saturated-fat diets and high cholesterol diets cause atherosclerotic lesions in monkeys. A selected group of monkeys were placed on such a diet for 5.4 years. After that time, half of the group was killed and examined and the other half was split into two groups again. The first group was placed on a low cholesterol diet. The remaining ones stayed on the diet high in saturated fats.

Plaque regression (plaque is the islands of hardened fat that gradually close arteries) was evaluated in one group of the survivors 2 years later and in the remaining monkeys 3.7 years later. Those who were sacrificed after 7 years had the same amount of scleroses as did those who were examined after 5 years.

The conclusion drawn from this was that, even after 10 years there was still significant plaque. Reducing plaque through dieting is slow and uncertain, the researchers concluded.

FISH OIL STOPS ATHEROGENICITY

It's been found that the consuming diets of juvenile African green monkey's which are enriched in n-6 poly unsaturated fats from birth have less coronary artery atherosclerosis than animals consuming diets rich in saturated fats. Plaque formation in the saturated fat diet group increased 28-fold between ages 32 months and 60 months. Animals on the unsaturated diet had a 7-fold increase in plaque in the same time period. The conclusion is that EFAs can be effective in decreasing the development of atherosclerosis.

FISHY DIETS

It's pretty well been established that small amounts of fish weekly has a protective effect against coronary heart disease in middle-aged people. A study presented in the International Journal of Epidemiology, April 1995, examined whether this was also true of the elderly. Coronary heart disease risk factors were measured in 272 people born before 1907 who were tracked for 17 years. The risk factors for fish eaters compared to non-fish eaters were highly significant. The outcome was that even small weekly amounts of fish protects the elderly as much as it does the middle-aged against heart disease.

ANOTHER IMPORTANT HELP TO AGING: *CHELATION THERAPY*

One theory of aging is that the body gradually accumulates too many toxic metals which stop the normal functioning of cells, or knocks them out of hormonal and neurological control. The other damage from toxic metals is to basic DNA. Genetic patterns can be disrupted as toxic metals catalyze oxidative reactions. Toxic metals make everything go wrong.

Where do they come from? Everywhere! The air, the water, but most often toxic metals come from the water we drink. Spring water as well as tap water contains suspended minerals so dispersed they are invisible. We need minerals, so that's good, only the ones found in our drinking water are not always the good ones.

The problem with *bad* minerals is they stick like glue once they get in. They find hiding places around the body, often in the bones or fat cells. They don't stay in their nest forever though; they slowly leach back out to clutter up enzyme systems and bring about serious problems such as Alzheimers disease.

The ONLY SUCCESSFUL way to rid the body of these menaces is to chelate them out. If you want to know more about chelation read "Bypassing the Bypass" or "The Chelation Way". Check your local book store for availability. Or you can contact me at the phone number listed in the back of the book.

ESSENTIAL OILS PLUS THE ANTIOXIDANT BETA CAROTENE

Antioxidants play a role in the prevention of coronary heart disease by inhibiting the peroxidation of polyunsaturated fatty acids. In this case, the antioxidant studied was beta carotene. The study included over 1,400 hundred patients in eight European countries. This study supports the idea that beta carotene plays a role in the protection of EFAs against oxidation and subsequently in the protection against heart attacks and cancer of the breast. The report appeared in the journal Atherosclerosis, Thrombosis, and Vascular Biology, June 95. As an aside, vitamin E did not seem to do the same.

I STRONGLY BELIEVE THAT <u>EVERY</u> OLDER PERSON SHOULD TAKE *CMO*. It is a natural substance, highly protective of good health. It is a substance that declines with age, I believe, and one that helps us fight off, or at least slow down the wear and tear of aging.

17

PROSTATE DISEASE

I'm confining my remarks in this section to prostatic enlargement because that's the only condition for which I have treating experience. It's very rare for a man to live a full life and avoid an enlarged prostate. If he hasn't developed an enlargement by his late fifties, he soon will. The many symptoms of prostate enlargement are so well known I will not recite all of them at this time.

I have picked several to focus on, though: urinary frequency, fatigue and sexual disinterest. This triad of symptoms flips a 180% on **CMO**. I was surprised to see how quickly a prostate gland could shrink. It can be as little time as a week. A second surprise was the complete disappearance of the other two symptoms I just mentioned.

CMO sometimes has a powerful aphrodisiac effect on men who haven't thought much about sex for some time. Some of them told me they could now perform twice a day.

LEONARD

This 58-year-old male was slowly developing chronic fatigue and anhedonia. Nothing was fun anymore, nothing in his life meant much either. After a long question and answer period I had no answers.

At this point it was tempting to write him off as depressed. But before we got to that possibility he remembered something he hadn't mentioned before, his enlarged prostate.

"Medications had not helped the swelling," he said. Neither had various nutritional items he had tried.

We talked about *CMO* and he agreed to give it a try.

All of his symptoms disappeared, within a week, in a rush of energy. In fact, he felt the *CMO* was pushing his energy a little too hard. He said it felt like a mild amphetamine. An exam showed a smaller gland.

"He had a new worry now," he said. The fear the prostate would enlarge again from overuse; he hadn't had so much sex since he was a kid. I told him it would certainly enlarge again if he kept up that kind of pace. He said he would just have to use more *CMO*.

RICHARD

Richard is in his sixties, he lifts weights every other day. He noticed some vague pains in his prostate during his workout. He said he felt a constant fullness in his pelvis, which got worse after sex. He was up two or three times a night to urinate, and once in a while, during his driving, he had to pull over to a gas station restroom. His PSA test was normal, but he worried about his prostate turning cancerous since his symptoms were so constant.

Just as Leonard did, Richard responded very quickly to *CMO*. Then he told me the same story Leonard had. A burst of energy, followed by a strong interest in sex. When I last talked to him he was asymptomatic. I told him to tame his urges or I'd see him back in my office again. He gave me a thumbs up and dashed off.

Another patient told me he was experiencing extreme orgasms the likes of which he'd never had before. This slowly died off after he discontinued the *CMO*. Because of this aphrodisia a number of people have asked if they could continue to use *CMO* indefinitely; I'll discuss this more in the last chapter.

If you were to ask me to list the top two diseases best served by *CMO* in the order of usefulness, I would list them this way: arthritis first and prostatic enlargement second. It may not work on everyone with prostate enlargement—what vitamin or drug does? But when it works—it's just grand.

ADDITIONAL AIDS

Prostada is a product of GERA VITA and quite helpful to the prostate. I have my patients take several capsules plus 50 mgs of zinc twice a day when they are on *CMO*. In most cases, their prostate returns to normal size within a week. I do not make any recommendations for the treatment of cancer pains.

18

PETS

CMO should be a fantastic find for pet owners. Just think how many times you've driven along a street and noticed a pet owner walking an old arthritic dog. Now that you know about *CMO*, next time you see them you might get the urge to pull over and tell them about *CMO*. I'm sure that owner would jump up and down to learn that their long-time companion would not suffer during the final year or two. The poor things will have an easier end at least.

CMO has been used on rats and humans with enormous success, so why not on pets? In fact *CMO* is a natural for pets because it is natural. As *CMO* is a product of nature, animals should take to it.

The only side effect of *CMO* for some pets, especially dogs, is constipation. The pet will have to be watched for this because it can make them very uncomfortable; enough for them to lie around and appear sick. Their stool may start out hard and discolored, then stop altogether.

The only answer is to see the veterinarian, or use a good

laxative while on **CMO**. Another answer is to spread the capsules over a longer period of time.

How many capsules should you give and how often? At this point, I can't say, I will have to defer to your veterinarian. If the doctor is uncertain, have him/her call KNOLLWOOD, Inc. listed in the back of the book.

I'm sorry to say I have only one case history for you. I used my own little dachsy for a test. She is getting older and X-rays show degeneration of the lower spine. She was taken to the veterinarian originally because she was sitting awkwardly, as though something was hurting. The veterinarian said there was nothing to be done, just to be careful with her activities. Since she was already a goner, according to the veterinarian, and it was only a matter of time before her back went, I decided to try **CMO**. I gave her one capsule daily. I didn't worry much about overdosing since her back was a bigger problem. I felt it was necessary considering the degree of damage she was facing.

She acted a little more active on the **CMO**, and had no symptoms, except for constipation. She had no bowel movements the last three days of the first week on **CMO** so I stopped the capsules. The next day I found a dozen mounds of stool around the back yard and a happy little rascal with a big smile on her face. She sits up normally now and doesn't appear in pain.

THE ESSENTIAL FATTY ACID CONNECTION AND PETS

Believe it or not there has been plenty of research to examine the use of EFAs for disease in pets. Pets have the same nutritional needs as humans, and develop deficiencies just as easily, especially when they have a chronic disease. Animals fed deficient vitamin E and selenium diets developed degenerative myopathy of the blood vessels and heart, for example.

Atopic disease has been greatly improved using essential oils: usually fish oil is used.

Dogs suffering from an atopic skin disease with extreme itching were treated with fish oil and most of them experienced major improvements.

In another experiment, fish oil allowed the reduction of prednisone during the treatment for skin diseases.

Cats fed evening primrose oil experienced a clearing of their dermatitis over a 12-week period when fish oil was added to their medical treatment. When the medicine and fish oil were combined, the two together produced a complete resolution of the dermatosis.

I've given you a few samples of the literature as a demonstration that essential oils are useful in the treatment of pet diseases. Since this is still an unexplored area, you may want to wait. I didn't, because I have no fear of **CMO**. I am certain it's a necessary nutrient for good health in all animals.

HEADACHES

There are three types of headaches that might respond to **CMO**: tension headaches, vasculitis, and the inflammatory type of migraines.

Let's take them one at a time.

TENSION HEADACHES

Many of these headaches are due to a painful neck or aching shoulders. This type of headache is almost always relieved by **CMO**. If the neck has some arthritis in it, that makes the likelihood of a response even better.

If the tension headache is caused by a required occupational postures, such as leaning over a desk during the work day, then **CMO** should help. If it's possible that the muscles in the neck are mildly inflamed, then **CMO** is worth trying.

Any subject whose previous symptoms improved on anti-inflammatory drugs or muscle relaxants is a prime candidate for **CMO**.

MIGRAINE HEADACHES

Sometimes it's almost impossible to differentiate between a migraine and a tension headache. Perhaps the two most important separating features are: pain that is confined to one side of the head, sometimes preceded by an aura, spots, light sensitivity or a visual disturbance. This doesn't happen with tension headaches. Migraine patients may be in so much pain they develop nausea and vomiting.

If you have had long-term headaches you may already have been accurately diagnosed. I say this tongue in cheek because numerous patients I see have had multiple diagnoses, and are still not sure what type of headache they have.

It's debatable whether migraines could be considered an actual inflammation although some types of migraine certainly appear to be. There have been anecdotal reports of *CMO* reversing migraines. I have not had such cases myself.

TEMPORAL ARTERITIS

The temples are a common area on the head for pain. Temporal arteritis is a syndrome with symptoms of temporal headaches, tenderness in the temporal area, and jaw pains. There may also be symptoms of polyarthralgia.

Vasculitis, which some doctors consider different from temporal arteritis, is characterized by inflamed blood vessels. It can affect any size vessel and any area of distribution.

To many people a headache may seem like a simple problem almost below the dignity of concern, whose treatment would surely be an easy task for a good doctor. The fact is that very few headaches seen by a doctor are solved in one visit. Hundreds of diseases start off with discomfort and headaches, and so the doctor has a lot of sorting to do.

CMO is not going to solve everyone's headache, but some people will benefit, just as others have.

At this point I can say that I have seen *CMO* improve tension-type headaches more than migraines.

ADDITIONAL AIDS

Ibuprofen cream is now available over the counter to be rubbed into the temples to relieve headaches. Many of my patients say it is not terribly effective. I have suggested they spread it out over a wider area which sometimes works.

I have used folic acid (four 800 mcg tablets) with each dose of *CMO*. Each individual has a different set of triggers for headaches and remedies which makes this one of the most difficult diseases to conquer. A perfect headache remedy for one individual may make your headache worse. This is the curse of the chronic headache sufferer.

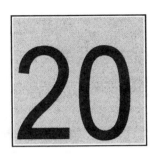

MENTAL ILLNESS

I don't know whether I should call this section mental illness or not, because I'm mostly going to touch on common problems like stress. But I will cover other states of mind like schizophrenia.

You are probably wondering why I would include this type of problem. I include it because I have seen some unusual responses to **CMO** that bear repeating. I also include it because of the essential fatty acid connection.

FISH OIL—EFAs

Since dietary intake of n-6 and n-3, essential fatty acids, influence the biophysical and biochemical properties of cell membranes, they do influence mental and emotional states. Epidemiological studies in various countries and in the U.S. in the last century suggest that decreased n-3 fatty acid consumption correlates with increased rates of depression. This is also consistent with a well-established positive correlation between depression and coronary artery disease.

Long chain n-3 polyunsaturated acid deficiency is known to contribute to depressive symptoms in alcoholism, MS and post partum depression.

The American Journal of Clinical Nutrition, July 1995, printed an article postulating EFAs as a viable treatment for depression. Some studies indicate it might be, because omega 6 fatty acid metabolism has been shown to be affected by stress.

Low EFA values might result from depletion of plasma stores for immunoregulatory prostenoids formation, or from modification of metabolic pathways by cortisol or other cytokine compounds implicated in stress. EFAs may be an important component of the physiological effects of psychological stress.

SCHIZOPHRENIA

Schizophrenics manifest a wide range of disturbing physical symptoms, such as, impaired sexual function, temperature control, low blood pressure, disrupted sleep patterns, excessive thirst, poor memory, insensitivity to pain, and chronic unhappiness.

Empirical research has demonstrated that plasma levels of essential fatty acids, glycoproteins and prostaglandins are abnormally low in the urine of schizophrenics.

The nervous system is the organ with the second greatest concentration of lipids. These lipids participate directly in membrane functioning. Brain development is genetically programmed. It is therefore necessary to ensure that nerve cells receive an adequate supply of nutrients, especially of lipids.

Scientists know that decreased levels of red blood cell EFAs in schizophrenic patients lie in an initial stage of an EFA pathway, possibly a defective uptake in the membranes of the red blood cells. Since fatty acid composition of membranes phospholipids affects the relative degree of membrane fluidity, it is suggested that these findings lend further support to the notion that RBC membrane dynamics are altered in schizophrenia.

When brain cells become deficient in EFAs, the speed of recuperation from these anomalies is extremely slow for brain cells, organelles, and microvessels, in contrast to other organs. A decrease in alpha-linolenic series acids in the membranes results in a 40% reduction in the metabolism of nerve terminals. Membrane fluidity is affected. Learning behavior is markedly altered. EFAs tend to resist certain neurotoxic agents such as lead.

The effects of polyunsaturated fatty acid deficiency have been extensively studied: prolonged deficiency leads to death in animals.

COLEY

I recently treated a patient with a dissociative disorder who had been having increasingly frequent auditory hallucinations: she heard a man's voice. The man's voice would come upon her suddenly when she was involved in some activity, jolting her. When she turned, no one was there. If she was busy and distracted when the voice appeared, she would answer without thinking, then catch herself. The "voice" was distinct and as loud as a real person, but the man was not threatening or sinister. The mysterious "voice" completely disappeared after one week of *CMO.* It did not return after she stopped *CMO.*

CMO has been a memory enhancer for some people, too. In another case of mine a patient was able to memorize the psychiatric DSM-4 manual during the week before her final exam.

Sometimes *CMO* improves conditions that do not really

have a name. One of these conditions is excessive thirst and urination of unexplained cause. The patient I'm thinking of has been examined by numerous doctors who have ruled out diabetes, kidney disease and all other possible causes, and, after extensive studies, did not offer her any form of treatment.

The female I'm describing urinates from two to three times the normal amount of urine daily, often over 5000 cc's. She has filled two and three 24-hour urine collection containers. This is not surprising because she drinks many gallons of water and beverages each day. Her symptom is a constant, overpowering thirst. Her mouth and throat are excessively dry, which indicates to me an overactive autonomic nervous system.

CMO returned this patient's thirst to normal within one day. During her entire *CMO* therapy she had normal urinary patterns. She did not visit the bathroom 4 and 5 times nightly as she had previously, and she was not starved for water. Unfortunately, this pattern returned when she stopped the *CMO*. I think it is imperative that we determine the safety of long-term use. See my discussion on this in the last chapter.

21

CETYL MYRISTOLEATE'S FRIENDS

This chapter is to provide you with a list of synergistic nutrients which will enhance the effects of **CMO**. If you were to ask me "Why do we need enhancers, isn't **CMO** enough?" I would have to answer that **CMO** has been extremely effective by itself, but it isn't perfect. That being the case, it's always prudent to build in a little extra insurance.

There are two more reasons for making these suggestions. First, all nutrients work better with coenzymes which are partners, or assistants. Secondly, **CMO** doesn't negatively interact with anything that we know of, so why not use therapeutic agents already known to improve the disease to be treated. You'll see better what I'm talking about as we get further into this chapter.

The five specific nutrients I'm going to be talking about are: the antioxidant; coenzyme Q10: the amino acids; taurine and carnatine, and the minerals; selenium and vanadyl sulfate.

I have been using **CMO** on patients for some time now and I frequently combine it with other nutrients to double its effect. For example, **CMO** is helpful for hypertension, but add the antioxidant superoxide desmutase (SOD) and you've doubled its power. That's the sort of thing I'm going to be talking about in this chapter. I have selected five nutrients that have been extensively studied by researchers, and there is no doubt they can reverse some diseases.

If **CMO** is pleased to receive a helping hand—what's wrong with that?

Think of it however you wish; the nutrients beef up **CMO**, or **CMO** makes each of them stronger. The important thing about all this is that readers have solid evidence that there are viable alternatives to drugs.

We must do all we can to overcome a serious disease. Sometimes we are fighting a disease and it's a matter of survival, cancer for example. Other times a disease makes us so miserable we just want to be done with it for the sake of our sanity. For these reasons and others, it's important to do everything we can to solve the problem. The use of multiple nutrients is no different from the use of multiple drugs.

The nutritional items I'm going to tell you about are known to be synergistic to fatty acids and to **CMO**. They strengthen them. And that's what we want, isn't it? We want the best nutrients we can get our hands on in the highest potency.

SELENIUM

Selenium is as friendly to **CMO** as it is to the EFAs. This metal ion defends the reservoir of EFAs in cerebral tissue against oxidation, which is very helpful if we are trying to slow aging. Rats given selenium were found to have higher levels of tissue EFAs.

In an Italian study, 53 women and 52 men from the village

of Nove, near Vicenza in northern Italy were interviewed to determine if there was a relationship between aging and three nutrients: selenium, vitamin A and E. Aging, the results showed, was associated with a progressive decline in selenium as well as a decline in EFAs.

Just a reminder that EFAs determine cellular membrane fluidity, which controls virtually everything that goes on inside the cell. EFAs also regulate neuronal transmission, which controls every function the brain performs. Now, you can see why it's very important that cerebral EFAs be guarded.

The oxidative system is the chief protector of EFAs, and one of the most important of these antioxidants is selenium. It is part of the glutathione molecule, whose purpose is to protect brain enzymes from oxidative stress.

Gradually declining selenium levels are part of the aging process. It's nature's way of snuffing out those who have used up their allotted genetic time.

In Chapter 16 I talked about using **CMO** to resist aging and the diseases of aging. I have taken **CMO** to resist my own aging process, and I have given it to others for the same reason. Fortunately, there are no symptoms to disappear, thus telling us **CMO** is working, so we must have a little leap of faith here. Minor changes can be seen though. For example, as you get a tad older, your neck doesn't turn right or left as far as it used to. Using **CMO**, the range of motion of the neck returns to normal. It's a small change, but a noticeable one that helps you know that **CMO** has been there.

The real purpose for taking **CMO** is to replace something I think the body needs—some, as yet, unrecognized nutrient the body has lost, something scientists have not discovered yet. Perhaps this book will start them down the road to the secrets of **CMO**.

VANADYL SULFATE

When I treat a diabetic I always add vanadyl sulfate along with **CMO**. Vanadyl is an insulin mimic which can exert an enormous effect on the stabilization of blood glucose levels. Especially in non-insulin-dependent diabetes mellitus (NIDDM).

Oral administration of vanadium salts to severely diabetic rats leads to a spectacular decrease of plasma glucose levels in spite of the insulin deficiency of the animals.

How does vanadyl work in the diabetic? Six NIDDM patients were given 100/mg of vanadyl for 3 weeks. Sugar disposal was better in the liver, the muscles and the rest of the body. After three weeks of vanadyl, treatment was stopped. Tissue levels of vanadyl lasted another 2 weeks and probably longer (it wasn't checked after it was discontinued).

The one problem with vanadyl, though, is poor absorption through the gut: the ion has trouble making it past the gut wall.

Vanadyl helps repair the complications of diabetes by normalizing blood sugar. In this way vanadyl protects the heart from the damages of diabetes. Vanadyl protects vascular reactivity from the destruction of diabetes. For example, treatment with vanadyl completely prevents increased responsiveness of our largest artery, the aorta, to adrenaline. Apparently the aorta is overresponsive in the diabetic, which causes hypertension and arteriosclerosis. This can be prevented by vanadyl.

As I just mentioned, vanadyl has some neat, long-term benefits. In a recent study, vanadyl tissue levels persisted for 16 weeks following withdrawal of it, so the authors concluded that it is effective for chronic therapy, and its prolonged use does not lead to the development of tolerance. The length of treatment was one year. Over this period of time there was a significant decrease in

overall weight. Vanadyl prevented overeating, excessive thirst, high cholesterol and cataract formation.
The dosage may be lessened over time.

Some people believe that excess insulin is the main cause for hypertension, others believe that insulin is actually anti-hypertensive, that the problem is insulin resistance. Correction of insulin resistance usually aids blood pressure control, and in addition may decrease the likelihood of cardiovascular risk associated with hypertension.

Rats who were hypertensive and hyperinsulinemic were selected for treatment with vanadyl sulfate. Blood pressure was decreased by 25 points at the end of the study.

Lastly, I should mention that vanadyl, like selenium, is a major player in resisting the ravages of oxidative stress; an aging and disease hazard. Review the experience of Rena in Chapter 11.

CARNATINE

Sometimes I add the amino acid carnatine to the *CMO* treatment, and when I do, I also add lysine, another amino acid that magnifies the effect of carnatine. Carnatine can be very helpful to muscle weakness, muscle aches, and malfunctioning nerves. Carnatine facilitated the repair of sciatic nerves in one experiment by improving nerve conduction velocity.

I gave carnatine to a case of trigeminal neuralgia (facial nerve damage), and the "sparkles" and "shooting pains" disappeared within a week. Carnatine has been successful in the treatment of symptomatic diabetic neuropathy too.

Carnatine is a strong detoxifier in that it ensures the elimination of xenobiotic substances. Maybe this is the reason it has a reputation for being a brain and central nervous system protector as well as a shield against myocardial infarctions (heart attacks).

When rats were injected with ammonia they had seizures and severe alterations of brain metabolism. If carnatine was given before the ammonia there were no symptoms.

Carnatine stops arrhythmias and raises HDL to boot.

You would have to be crazy not to want a companion like carnatine on *CMO*'s side. *CMO* is powerful, but add another powerful nutrient, such as carnatine, and you double the chances of success.

I have seen carnatine reverse arrhythmias and raise HDL levels.

When I personally take carnatine, it upsets my stomach to such a degree I have to take food with it. Others have told me the same. I know of no other side effect.

TAURINE

If you think carnatine is great, wait till you hear about the amino acid taurine. It's a terrific friend of *CMO*.

It could be a great helper in the treatment for emphysema, because taurine plus niacin halt the progression of fibrosis, part of the degenerative process of emphysema.

Taurine is helpful to diabetics, altering carbohydrate metabolism in such a way that it lowers blood sugar by increasing the tissue's utilization of glucose. At the same time it is acting somewhat like insulin, it is facilitating insulin. Like vanadyl sulfate, taurine is a weaker version of insulin. Taurine helps the liver make more sugar and store it, which means it's also useful for the hypoglycemic.

Taurine blocks the progressive nerve fiber degeneration caused by diabetes. It has neurotrophic actions which counteract the hyperexcitability and pain seen in early diabetic neuropathy.

I always use taurine when I treat hypertensives, because it blocks peripheral serotonin, a powerful vasoconstrictor.

Taurine interferes with smooth muscle contraction so well that it has been used with some success in asthma.

The most important way taurine improves hypertensive status is to desensitize the overactive arterial walls of the larger blood vessels.

ALPERT

This older male was taking several blood pressure medicines when I first saw him, but his family doctor was thinking of prescribing them. The blood pressure was borderline—stress would send his blood pressure higher; I started him on *CMO*, taurine, and gave him a new diet.

Slowly, his systolic blood pressure fell but, best of all, his lower, diastolic levels below 90 fairly rapidly. It was a simple case and yet an important step in prevention. Had he started on the drug merry-go-round he might never have gotten off.

Taurine reduces blood lipids by reducing the absorption of dietary cholesterol and enhancing the breakdown of cholesterol. If you add niacin to the taurine, the effect is even stronger. Taurine is known to clear fatty livers by mobilizing the fats stored there.

This amino acid has membrane-stabilizing effects on cardiovascular tissue so it has been successful as an anti-arrhythmic nutrient. Taurine does this by blunting the plasma adrenaline levels. This reduces the oversensitive tissues throughout the vascular tree. At the same time, taurine reinforces the strength in the left ventricle of the heart at the same time. Three grams of taurine a day for six weeks has been known to turn congestive heart failure around.

COENZYME Q 10

Coenzyme Q 10 is a giant among nutrients, yet it is not appreciated and is under-utilized by most nutritionists. I hope I can bring its true value to light by the end of this chapter.

Coenzyme Q 10 is an amazing antioxidant with multiple uses the same as those nutrients mentioned in the previous chapter. I am going to limit the discussion to only two of its many uses: hypertension and cancer.

If you were to stand **CMO** next to coenzyme Q 10, **CMO** would be taller and have a longer reach, but coenzyme Q 10 would be right up there with it.

HYPERTENSION

Quite a number of studies have proven that coenzyme Q 10 can retract hypertension. In the Italian study by Digiesi et al, 26 patients with essential hypertension were given 50 mgs of coenzyme Q 10 twice a day for ten weeks. At the end of 10 weeks systolic blood pressure had dropped 18 points, from an average of 164 to an average 146. Diastolic blood pressure dropped an average of 12 points: 98 to 86.

At the same time the blood pressure was dropping so was the cholesterol: 223 average to 213. The HDL (good cholesterol) rose from an average of 41 to 43.

A second group of 11 patients were given the same routine and experienced almost an identical outcome. In discussing the results researchers noted that 30% of those in the study started it with abnormally low blood levels of coenzyme Q 10.

Coenzyme Q 10 levels can be lowered by aerobic training, hyperthyroidism and the therapeutic use of antihypertensive medications of the HMG-CoA reductase inhibitors class.

Another study was undertaken in Tyler, Texas by Langsjoen et al. This study was set up to attain a coenzyme Q 10 target blood level of 2.0 mcg/ml.

Fifty percent of the patients discontinued one to three blood pressure medicines by the end of the fourth month. Only 3% failed to respond favorably. At least 40% of the patients had a significantly favorable cardiac improvement in left ventricle strength. There were no interactions with the medications used for hypertension.

109 patients were studied whose average age was 62. It was interesting that the blood pressure didn't really begin to change until around the third month. When it started down it kept going.

Remember that all of these patients were on one to three hypertensive medicines when they started, so the starting blood pressure reflects what it was *during* treatment. The ending blood pressure relates to less hypertensive medications, or **no** medications. Systolic blood pressure dropped from an average of 159 to 147, and diastolic blood pressure dropped from 94 to 85.

The average time it took to drop at least one hypertensive medication was 4 months. Six of the 109 starting patients were not on medicines. Blood pressures of all 6 returned to normal. If you are just beginning to show signs of hypertension, it would be smart to start these nutrients right away. About 30% of those in the study ended up sans medicines. The researchers thought that coenzyme Q 10 was energizing the entire cardiovascular system, bringing it back to normal. Essential hypertension, in their view, was an adaptation of the cardiovascular system to an impairment of myocardial bioenergetics.

Another study was done in 1991 by Montaldo et al. Fifteen hypertensive patients were given 100 mgs of coenzyme Q 10 daily for 12 weeks. There was a significant drop in blood pressure and the heart was strengthened.

Just as an aside, a study by Knapp, "Fatty Acids and Hypertension", found that fish oil will also lower blood pressure.

CANCER

CMO may be useful for the suppression of pain in cancer patients. I have not used it for this purpose but it has possibilities. I would combine it with coenzyme Q 10, which has significant anti-cancer qualities. Both of these nutrients would be used complementary to standard medical treatments, of course.

The studies you are about to read prove beyond any doubt that coenzyme Q 10 is supportive of standard cancer therapy. I believe the same is true of *CMO*. Some individuals have already tried *CMO* for cancer, along with their traditional medical therapies. The information that I received was that a patient with cancer of the lungs and another with cancer of the breast had hard evidence of slowing cancer growth.

I'm not suggesting that **CMO** be used as a treatment for cancer: there is no evidence it would be of value, but it might be useful as a pain suppresser.

BREAST CANCERS REVERSED BY COENZYME Q 10

Let's take a look at how coenzyme Q 10 has bolstered the resistance of breast cancer patients.

The journal, Molecular Aspects of Medicine, published an article in 1994 entitled, "Apparent Partial Remission of Breast Cancer in 'High Risk' Patients Supplemented with Nutritional Antioxidants, Essential Fatty Acids, and Coenzyme Q 10". Lockwood, Maesgaard, Hanioka and Folkers were the researchers.

Folkers, perhaps the most experienced of the authors of this study, had conducted a previous study on coenzyme Q 10 and cancer plus a survey of thirty years of research pertaining to the subject.

The study consisted of thirty-two patients with breast cancer, ages 32 to 81. The cancer had already spread to the axillary nodes (underarm area) of this group, which is the reason they were called high risk.

The treatment consisted of taking a measured amount of coenzyme Q 10, and continuing their standard medical treatments concurrently.

The study lasted 18 months, during which they were supposed to take daily supplements of Vitamin C: 2850 mgs; Vitamin E: 2500 iu; B-carotene: 32.5 iu; selenium 387 micrograms: plus secondary vitamins and minerals. They also took essential fatty acids and coenzyme Q 10: 90 mgs per day. It is thought that these items synergize each other.

The recorded parameters during the treatment period were laboratory biochemical markers, clinical observations, tumor spread, and quality of life.

None of the women on coenzyme Q 10 were excused from their other scheduled therapies: surgery, radiology, chemotherapy and tamoxifen, etc., during the 18 months. Blood was tested periodically for coenzyme Q 10 levels, to be sure the subjects complied with the routine. At the end of the first year, their blood levels of coenzyme Q 10 averaged a rise from 0.82 mg/l. at the start to 1.60 mg/l. at the end of 12 months. Beta-carotene levels went up from 838 to 2862. Vitamin E changed from 11.3 at the beginning to 33.4, B 6 from 30 to 641, Selenium from 138 to 547. As you can see, even with what I would call modest doses of vitamins and minerals, the blood was saturated with nutrients.

All of the other minerals—calcium, magnesium, manganese, zinc, iron, copper and lithium—stayed the same.

Natural killer cell counts went up from 207 to 253 and lymphocyte cells (white blood cells) went from 1355 to 1894.

The interesting thing about these findings was that their starting level of coenzyme Q 10 was 0.82 mg/l. which is well below an average person's blood level of 1.45 mg/l. It took 90 days for this to rise, but it kept going up. The highest level anyone reached was 2.81 mg/l. Studies have shown that normal, non-cancerous individuals would have faster and higher rises than these patients experienced.

None of the patients died during the trial! That was the most important observation of the study. No one in this group showed any signs of further distant metastases either. Weight was not lost and requests for pain medications declined significantly. *Full remissions occurred in six of the patients!*

There were no side effects during the treatment.

All of these amazing changes occurred in spite of the admission by the research team that the 90 mg dose they were giving was still too low for adequate response.

CASE 1

One of the patients, a 64-year-old female, had verified metastases to the 10th thoracic vertebra. She began the study taking 520 mgs of morphine daily and ended the program on 1000 mg of aspirin twice daily and no morphine. This patient had had a double mastectomy five years previous to this study, but her cancer had progressed slowly from that time.

However, during this program there was no further progression, as confirmed by bone scanning.

CASE 2

This is a 52 year-old-woman who entered the program in serious clinical condition. She had had a mastectomy one year prior to this trial but the cancer came back. Tumor cells were found in her pleural fluid and breast cancer in her X-rays.

A few weeks after she entered the trial her clinical condition significantly improved. X-rays showed the pleural fluid had disappeared and the lung cancer was gone.

CASE 3

A 70-year-old woman had a lobular carcinoma in the right breast, as determined by biopsy. A mastectomy was performed but they missed some of the cancer. Another biopsy was taken after the coenzyme Q 10 trial and the tumor bed was completely free of tumor tissue.

CASE 4

An 82-year-old had a breast removed eight years before this trial. They found a ductile carcinoma, grade 2, with metastases to the axillae, and infiltration of the tumor into nerves on both sides of the breast.

She entered the study with numerous metastases around her surgical scar. During the treatment with coenzyme Q 10, the metastases disappeared, the axillary lymph nodes became non-palpable, and the patient appeared to be in excellent health.

CASE 5

A 54-year-old lady had a mastectomy to remove a carcinoma in her right breast. She came into the trial just before beginning chemotherapy. In reviewing the case it was concluded that coenzyme Q 10 had allowed her to tolerate the chemotherapy well, with no hair loss, and to recover without incident.

The final outcome of this trial was:

1. None of the patients died during the study.
2. At least few would have died, statistically speaking, if they had not been taking coenzyme Q 10.
3. No one lost weight.
4. Those on painkillers reduced their doses.
5. There was no further spread of the cancers. There were no side effects except for some yellowing of the palms in a few, due to the beta-carotene.
6. At the end of the test the research staff recommended that the dose of coenzyme Q 10 be raised to 300 mg daily.

This research group recontacted all of the patients again six months after the trial had ended, and found that the condition of the 32 patients had not changed significantly. No one had died. The two patients who had increased their dose of coenzyme Q 10 to 390 mgs daily, had complete remissions of their cancers, which had been medically verified.

Even though the above research was done exclusively on coenzyme Q 10, I consider *CMO* to be just as powerful. Think of the possibilities of the two together.

The above study was based on the National Research

Council's scientific survey in which it had found an association between diet and cancer. This information is important to know because one out of every five deaths in this country is caused by cancer.

Breast cancer alone causes more deaths in women 40 to 44 than any other disease.

NUTRITION, DIET AND CANCER

The differences in the frequencies of various cancers seem to be related to differences in diets. Hormones make some difference but diet is considered more important.

In his 1990 epidemiological study, Dneckt, et al. found an 11 times higher risk of breast cancer when the diet was low in foods containing selenium and vitamin E.

A number of other nutritional supplements—Vitamin A, beta carotene and selenium, for example, have also been found to have anti-cancerous benefits. In 1987, Van der Merwe, et al. reported marked improvements in most of 21 patients being supplemented with gamma-linolenic acid who had untreatable malignancies.

COENZYME Q 10, NUTRITION AND CANCER

An extensive review of the literature on vitamin and nutritional entities and their relationship to the prevention and treatment of cancer produced more than 200 references of the successful treatment of cancer using coenzyme Q 10.

Folkers, one of the members of this research team, had previously used Coenzyme Q 10 in another treatment study. Three of the subjects in the study had cancer, four had heart disease and one had diabetes: all of them responded positively to coenzyme Q 10 during the 96-day trial.

Folkers, however, found that the dose of 60 mgs daily which he was using at the time was too small. He discovered another thing too. Coenzyme Q 10 seems to require the assistance of a number of cofactors (nutritional aids) to be fully effective.

Vitamin Q 10 has been found to stimulate the defense system for resistance to infections such as viral, bacterial and protozoal. It also defended against senescence and to chemically-induced cancers.

ANOTHER TRIAL FOR BREAST CANCER

Karl Folkers, along with Lockwood and Maesgaard, published another paper in 1994 on the treatment of breast cancer with coenzyme Q 10. They called it "Partial and Complete Regression of Breast Cancer in Relation to Dosage of Coenzyme Q 10."

CASE 1

The patient was a 59-year-old female with a family history of breast cancer. In 1991, the patient was operated on for a tumor in the left breast. A mammography done two months later showed the existence of a malignant tumor. A mammography in May 1992 indicated a widespread tumor in the left axillae. The patient had been on 90 mg. daily of coenzyme Q 10 since 1991, but it apparently hadn't been enough. The dose was raised by 300 mgs daily, to 390 mgs daily.

In November of 1993, the tumor could no longer be felt in the breast or under the arm. A mammography in December, 1993, again showed no signs of a tumor.

Encouraged by the first case, the authors repeated their protocol on a second case.

CASE 2

A 74-year-old female was first seen in September of 1993. She had a small node where the breast enters the right axilla. It was found to be cancerous on removal, however, some of the cancer still remained.

She was placed on 300 mgs of coenzyme Q 10 in October of 1993. On January 25, 1994, a physical examination and mammography revealed no sign of cancer. As of February 1995, the patient was still on coenzyme Q 10 and still free of cancer.

Dr. Lockwood, one of the authors of this paper, has seen 200 new breast cancers per year for 35 years and admits he had never seen a spontaneous regression of a 2.0 cm breast tumor before, and has never seen a comparable regression on any conventional anti-tumor therapy.

CONCLUSIONS

Bearing in mind what you have just read, the one thing certain is that nutritional supplements can have major impacts on the body's ability to repair itself. *CMO*, which I believe may be as powerful as coenzyme Q 10, can be combined with it to make a dynamic duo.

I would never in a thousand years suggest you use *CMO* in place of standard medical care, especially when it comes to cancer. You *MUST* stay with the treatment prescribed by your personal physician, by all means. Before starting you must discuss all of your plans with your treating physician, and let him make the decision.

ORAL TOLERIZATION

This chapter is an attempt to explain how **CMO** works. There are a number of theoretical possibilities. Is it an oral tolerizer, a surfactant, a vitamin cofactor, a newly discovered essential fatty acid or maybe even something else?

Let's go through the possibilities one at a time.

ORAL TOLERIZATION

Technically, this area of science is called "the field of cellular immunology", or "the field of immunoregulation." It has to do with your body's ability to decide what is YOU and what is not YOU.

Your white blood cells are part of your immune system and the source of autoimmune problems. If you become infected they fight off the invader. They have no eyes though, so they depend on chemical signals to decide what is YOU and what is not. The special group of white blood cells that make this decision are called the T lymphocytes.

It can be dangerous if they make a mistake and decide

that a part of YOU is a foreign substance. Not being perfect, they make mistakes like this millions of times. Over 20 million people in this country have autoimmune diseases. No one knows for sure what starts them. Most likely it's a set of unfortunate circumstances all happening at the same time. Usually it happens at a time when your immune system is compromised from fatigue or stress.

We treat this disease by administering immuno-suppressive vaccines, which fall into two categories: the preventative mode or the curative mode. That is, whether the vaccine is given before or after one has been exposed to the disease. In the case of *CMO* we are in the curative mode, that is we are taking it after we are already highly sensitized to the antigen. A person unexposed to an antigen (antigens are substances which can stimulate the body to produce antibodies—a pollen, a food, etc.) is said to be both cellularly and molecularly naive.

The typical T cell defense response starts with IgM antibody production, followed some days later by massive production of IgG, IgA, and IgE (IgE is associated with allergy). These antigens can be repeatedly boosted upwards by further injections of antigens.

None of the prior attempts to desensitize IgM, IgG and IgE have substantially down-regulated antibody production once a persistent immune response, generated by repeated doses of immunogen, is established.

Antihistamines have nothing to do with how antibodies are made or not made, so this form of chemotherapy is purely palliative. Oral tolerization researchers are looking for a cure to the disease, not symptom relief. They are searching for an antigen, just like the one that caused the trouble but a nontoxic one that can turn the sensitized system off. They are looking for a vaccine that will be a long-lasting suppresser of the reaction.

The most pressing reason why this approach is being studied is the increasing failure of other therapies.

It may be that somehow this form of treatment is restoring a natural balance that should have kept its place, but didn't: a homeostatic balance between stimulatory and suppressive forms of antigenic materials.

The most important factor that determines the balance seems to be the physical size and charge on the protein antigen.

What we need it a final state of non-reactivity to an antigen. We need something that will limit the unchecked proliferation of cells that make antigens after exposure to the antigen. We need immunological paralysis (paralysis = tolerance).

Oral tolerization is a form of molecular therapy and not pharmaceutical therapy. It consists of imparting the ability to down regulate the persistent production of antibodies, using a suppressive form of antigen. This, when it is fully developed and in place, will be a powerful therapeutic tool to avoid toxic nonspecific chemotherapies.

It turns out that small antigens are the suppressers and large molecular antigens are the bad guys, the stimulators. Tiny antigens will not stimulate antibody response no matter how much of the antigen is present. These little ones are extremely potent, and can inhibit the immune response to the larger antigens.

Under normal exposure, an antigen will attach itself to a white blood cell called a B cell, triggering it's transformation into a plasma cell, which can then pump out antibodies.

When small antigens are present things go differently. These spoilers competitively steal receptors from the larger antigens.

By attaching themselves to B lymphocytes (the cells most

sensitive to stimulation) they interfere with their big brothers who could have easily set off reactions. The little antigens do not set off reactions, however.

When the antigen is a food it eventually reaches special lymphoid tissue in the gut called "peyer's patches". This is where immune reactions start. These gut cells migrate and interact with other cells, all of which end up in antibody production.

These tiny antigens in *low doses* actively suppress antigen production. If they are given in high doses they produce clonal energy: another way to inactivate antibody production.

In one study, treatment antigens were placed on a polymer carrier, a molecular platform. When the polymer is swallowed it combines with specific antibodies, and becomes an *immune complex* which is recognized by the Kupffer cells in the liver as rubbish, and is removed from the blood. This process is called phagocytosis, breakdown and excretion.

This removal process can last for several days or be as short as 12 hours. Under normal circumstances, a group of specialized cells, called plasma cells, would replenish the antibody supply if it were depleted. The plasma cells themselves must also be replenished from an activated B cell population. This replacement will not occur with the oral tolerization curative process. Instead, the serum levels of specific IgM and IgE declined.

A 2 mg dose of suppressive polymer (an unusually large dose) is necessary to overcome the preexisting high levels of antibodies in boosted mice. The reason why is that a very large proportion of a given polymer is immediately taken out of the blood by the Kupffer cell in the liver, so only a small fraction of the polymer stays in the circulation long enough to do its work. Such removal from circulation may be enhanced by immune complex formation, which occurs soon after the suppressive polymer's injection.

The biggest advantage to this curative process is its sustained effects. It turns out that the plasma cell numbers (the white blood cells that manufacture antibodies) are semi-permanently suppressed. Therefore, there are fewer of them to make antibodies. They are actually the targets for the suppressive polymers, which is exactly what we want to happen.

It is thought that the B-cell precursors of plasma cells are more likely to be a target of antigen specific suppression. The end result is some kind of a long-lasting functional depletion of the B cells, the mothers of the plasma cells. B cells then are either inactivated or left almost nonexistent.

It's a real blessing that oral tolerance can be induced at any age, young or old.

MULTIPLE SCLEROSIS

Let me repeat the definition of oral tolerization in case you've forgotten; it is the oral administration of antigens (a specially selected food), which causes a state of immunologic unresponsiveness.

Multiple sclerosis is thought to be caused by T lymphocytes that recognize myelin sheaths around nerves as being foreign substances. In MS, myelin basic protein and proteolipid protein are the targets of the T cell overactivity, an autoimmune reaction.

Perivascular infiltration of mononuclear cells into the central nervous system (white blood cells gathering around nerves in the central nervous system) is a pathologic hallmark for MS. The white blood cells that collect around nerves are CD4+ cells, T-cells and macrophages. Although various cells in the central nervous system are capable of cytokine production, the expression of these cytokines is localized around the inflammatory infiltrates.

Let me define a cytokine before we go on. Cytokines are proteins that are secreted to cause inflammation and proliferation of white blood cells. There are four groups of them: (IL) interleukins, (TNF) tumor necrosis factor, interferons and hematopoietic growth factors.

Multiple sclerosis is a central nervous system autoimmune inflammation. Immune suppression has been the main therapeutic approach so far because of the overwhelming evidence that immune system overactivity is behind MS.

The majority of drugs used for MS are highly toxic and not really specific. The same conditions are also true of type one diabetes, and rheumatoid arthritis. The goal is to develop a more specific and less toxic approach to the treatment.

THE HARVARD STUDY

In the Harvard study, 30 individuals with relapsing-remitting MS received daily capsules of bovine myelin to determine the oral tolerization effect to myelin antigens. 12 out of 15 had an attack in the control group, but only 6 out of 15 in the myelin-treated group. T cells reactive to myelin basic protein dropped significantly in the treated group. The oral administration of antigens induces a state of immunologic unresponsiveness, and that's what we want. There were no side effects.

In this study 300 mgs of bovine myelin were given daily for a year to 15 individuals and a placebo to 15 others with MS. None of the 8 males in the myelin-treated group had an attack. After the study ended the male patients in the treated group remained on the myelin for a total of two and a half years. During this time their disease remained stabilized with no attacks.

Oral administration of MBP suppresses MS-like symptoms, and this is mediated by CD8+ cells and T-cells that transfer protection.

When myelin basic protein was given there was a marked reduction of the accumulation of white blood cells and a reduction of all inflammatory cytokines. The results of this study indicate that suppression of the MS symptoms either induced by oral tolerization or that which occurs during natural recovery is related to the secretion of inhibitory cytokines or factors that actively suppress the inflammatory process in the target organ.

RHEUMATOID ARTHRITIS

Rheumatoid arthritis is an inflammatory synovial disease thought to be caused by T cells reacting to an antigen within the joint. The most likely antigen is type 2 collagen, which is the major protein in articular cartilage. Oral tolerization works in animal models, so it was tried on human volunteers, in a study by Wang et al.

Chicken type 2 collagen was manufactured for the study. 60 patients with severe rheumatoid arthritis ingested the collagen for 3 months. Four of the patients had complete remissions, and none of the patients experienced side effects.

The article starts by admitting that current treatments are inadequate in that they only partially control the rheumatoid arthritis. It is also admitted that the side effects of the drugs make them dangerous for long-term use. The ideal therapy would reduce the symptoms without the toxicity.

CONCLUSIONS

Is *CMO* a suppressing form of antigen? The closest correlation to this in terms of treatment response, is that *CMO* is extremely effective against rheumatoid arthritis, a known autoimmune disease. *CMO's* effect seems to be lasting, often a two week treatment lasts for years. Oral tolerization antigens usually require years of use by contrast, but they keep the disease in check.

Myelin basic protein is just what it says—it's a protein. *CMO*, on the other hand, is a fatty alcohol. Some scientists think *CMO* will fit into the autoimmune grid somehow. Overall there might be some connection between *CMO* and the oral tolerization approach, but research will have to decide.

Rheumatoid arthritis responds to other nutrients, but they seldom maintain the kind of improvements that come from *CMO* or the oral tolerization techniques. The tendency for the disease not to recur after treatment is the one major feature that strongly points toward oral tolerization as the underlying curative mechanism for *CMO*.

24

IS CMO A SURFACTANT?

NATURES HARD/SOFT BALANCE

CETYL MYRISTOLEATE is an anionic surfactant and one of its effects on the body is to soften tissues hardened by cholesterol. Cholesterol is the starch of the body, stiffening cells so they can keep their shape, somewhat like a flexible cartilage would. This soft/hard consistency is an important balance in nature. Think about it: the structure of a cell can't be a plate of mush, it has to have plasmature. Metabolic factors, on the other hand, can't move around in cell membranes if they are dense as tree sap. Young, healthy tissues are supple while chronic disease tends to produce leathery tissues.

Nature uses *surfactant oils* such as the EFAs to break up log jams, at least that's the way it's supposed to work. *Surfactant oils* make the cell walls more permeable and flexible, which is appropriate for healthy cellular functions.

CMO may very well be a powerful *immune modulator* as

suspected by doctors using it, but its most powerful effect, I suspect, is as a **surfactant**. A LUBRICANT—SOMETHING AKIN TO WD 40. It actually softens aged tissues, fading age spots at the same time. The amazing thing is how fast it works. *CMO* unfreezes the bound tissues overnight, as would WD 40.

FATTY DEGENERATION

Fatty degeneration may be the bind that *CMO* dissolves. Fat droplets are seen in muscle cells of rheumatoid arthritis and that is the only difference between rheumatic and normal cells. These fat globules are large enough, and there seems to be enough of them, to deform the cell. Swelling stretches the pain fibers enough to set off pain.

The fat droplets just described are saturated and underactive, so they can't take part in the cell's metabolism. We call these pockets of oil, "Fatty Degeneration". When there are enough fat deposits to interfere with normal biological functions we say the tissue or organ is suffering from fatty degeneration. Fatty degeneration can occur in any organ system—arteries, liver, joints. . . anywhere. Even the heart can be a site of fatty degeneration.

Atherosclerosis can be defined as deposits of fatty material in arteries, so atherosclerosis might even be called fatty degeneration. Most such deposits are made up of cholesterol, which is one of the stickiest and hardest substances around.

Sclerotic plaques of fat make the contour of the artery such that it encourages aggregations of cells and clots.

Unsaturated fatty acids are slick, able to keep the sticky fatty acids (saturated fats) separated—that's why alternative care doctors and nutritionists urge people to use EFAs.

Gummy platelets also develop when the diet is high in the

wrong foods. Just as too many sticky (saturated) fats are bad for you, *too few* slick fatty acids (EFA) are also bad for you.

The order of viscosity might go something like this, with hardeners at the top.

Rancid fats
Saturated fatty acids
Cholesterol
Vegetable oils
Flax seed and evening primrose oil
Fish oils
CETYL MYRISTOLEATE is at the bottom.

Now let's suppose that **CMO** is a *super thinner*. It is then so powerful that it could soften and dissolve some of the fatty areas around the joint, allowing tendons and tissues to slide back and forth easily. It also acts as an immune paralyzer, reducing the accumulation of white blood cells in and around the joints. This is totally logical since affected joints reduce in size rapidly. As the swelling subsides, the hands move around less painfully: they seem more lubricated. The inflammation disappears because oils are soothing to red, angry tissue.

INFLAMMATION

We can't fully discuss inflammation without defining what we mean by cytokine, one of the key factors in inflammation.

Cytokines are proteins that are secreted to cause inflammation and proliferation of white blood cells. There are four groups: (IL) interleukins, (TNF) tumor necrosis factor, interferons and hematopoietic growth factors. Cytokines have a particularly important action on vascular walls. This is especially important to the generation of atherosclerosis. Cytokine-releasing cells also cause coagulation. Cytokines make the walls of arteries so sticky that white blood cells adhere and cause damage. They also cause cellular walls in tissues and blood vessels to be more permeable, allowing arteries and veins to leak fluids.

The cytokines and eicosanoids just mentioned are not the bad guys until they go too far. When they overdo it they become fire bugs. We call them pyrogenic (fire starters). Fire starters can be blocked by cortisone.

Usually what sets off the firestarters is exposure to a toxin or invading microorganism. The resulting inflammation destroys the threat.

Cytokines increase both sides of the balance, playing good guy/bad guy, involving themselves in both oxidant production as well as antioxidant defenses.

The following nutrients have been proven to reduce inflammation in joint diseases, acute and chronic pancreatitis, and respiratory distress syndrome: copper, zinc, selenium, N-acetylcysteine, cysteine, methionine, taurine, and vit E.

EFAs AND INFLAMMATION

An inflammation is one of the body's defenses against an infection or a toxin. There is also a balance in this process of defending oneself, as there is in all of the bodily processes. The balance is to produce just enough inflammation to defend, but not too much. A strong torch can burn off an attacker, but too hot a flame can burn down the host. . . us.

The EFAs that cause inflammation are called omega 6, also referred to as n-6. The EFAs that reverses inflammation are called omega 3's, often referred to as n-3's.

N-6 EFAs are structurally important for cell membranes, they act as precursors for arachidonic acid (AA), and the eicosanoids: prostaglandins, thromboxanes and leukotrienes. These factors are also related to inflammations and hardening of tissues.

Rheumatoid arthritis, inflammatory bowel disease and impaired immune competence such as occurs with burns, post-op stress and coronary angioplasty aftereffects, are examples of inflammations that are out of control. N-6 EFAs are counter-balanced by the n-3 EFAs. If not counter-balanced, the n-6s will produce exaggerated effects in acute stress responses causing immunosuppression, platelet aggregation and excessive or chronic inflammation. N-3 EFAs act as precursors of complementary eicosanoids which counteract the exaggerated responses of arachidonic acid-derived eicosanoids.

N-3 requirements can be covered by weekly consumption of 3 portions of fatty fish. The British nutritional foundation recommends a daily intake of 3-4 gms of standardized fish oil a day.

FATTY ALCOHOLS

CMO is a fatty alcohol, biochemically speaking. Fatty alcohols do have immunological effects. Another similar fatty acid, n-hexacosanol, has been shown to exert pronounced effects on central neurons. It promotes the survival of injured cholinergic neurons, thus it could be useful in diseases involving neuronal degenerations. Long chain fatty acids like this are generally endowed with immunosuppressive properties.

Myristic acid is a non-essential fatty acid which does have a strong effect on potassium channels throughout the cells. Potassium channel openers are the base of a relatively new group of drugs that are just being developed.

COULD *CMO* BE STIMULATING ADENOSINE RECEPTORS?

The acute anti-inflammatory effects of methotrexzte are mediated, at least in part, by increased extracellular adenosine concentrations at inflamed sites. This observation suggests that other agents that increase extracellular adenosine might also reduce inflammation. The development of agents that promote adenosine release at sites of inflammation is a novel strategy for the treatment of inflammatory diseases such as rheumatoid arthritis.

CMO could logically stimulate these receptors as part of its overall effects on the body.

Adenosine receptors are present on most cells and organs. Adenosine inhibits many of the functions of white cells: phagocytosis, generation of toxic oxygen metabolites, and adhesion. Unfortunately, it does not inhibit degranulation or chemotaxis. Recent studies indicate that nonmetabolized adenosine receptor stimulants are potent anti-inflammatory agents. Is *CMO* one of them?

WHAT DOES THE INVENTOR OF *CMO* THINK ABOUT IT'S MECHANISMS?

Mr. Diehl, the discoverer of *CMO,* admits he has no clue as to how it works, and nearing ninety, he couldn't care less.

CMO has broad spectrum effects which mimic other substances. I have already alluded to its similarity to the EFAs and to oral tolerizers (anti-autoimmune effects). We know it has surfactant effects. The most common statement heard by all of the users is, "I feel freed up and so much looser."

CMO may be an anti-oxidant and a circulatory enhancer. It's also somewhat like adenosine, capsiscin and cortisone. All of these biochemicals are anti-inflammatory and pain-relieving and so are similar to *CMO.*

25

IS STANDARD MEDICAL CARE
A LONG-TERM OPTION?

Drugs are here to stay—and that's a reality. A second reality is that drugs can seriously _harm people_. And a third reality is that safe substitutes for drugs are sorely needed.

You might conclude that I'm opposed to drugs by the time you reach the end of this chapter—I'm not. I just think we should be open to alternatives.

This chapter covers the side effects of current drugs used for the treatment of arthritis and other diseases. The emphasis will be on NSAIDs (non-steroid anti-inflammatory drugs) and methotrexate. I'm not discussing the side effects of cortisone because you already know them.

The anti-rheumatic drugs are basically anti-inflammatory, and, therefore, are the centerpieces of treatment for all chronic diseases.

This chapter is to remind those who have become temporarily comfortable with these drugs that _all of them_ have long-term dangers. In fact, when you consider you may spend a life time with drugs, the treatment is almost worse than the disease. It doesn't seem so on a day-to-day basis because current pain and swelling are being controlled, which is paramount to someone who is miserable and incapacitated. Down the line, when one's liver or kidney fails, the truth emerges.

As an example, the British Journal of Rheumatology reported in 1995 that anti-inflammatory drug users frequently develop chronic renal (kidney) impairment and renal (kidney) papillary necrosis (tissue death).

The statistics will vary, but it could be as many as one out of five users who suffer kidney failure. That means 20% of those on NSAIDs risk a fatal illness. An important risk, to say the least.

The anti-inflammatories, NSAIDs, and cortisone are also known to cause osteoporosis (bone thinning). This may make the original disease worse because it can be the cause of fractures, especially compression fractures of the vertebrae.

You've seen these people with compression fractures, they are shorter and hunched over. 58% of the women using these drugs suffer similar consequences to some degree.

But none of this is really new. Everyone knows that medicines, used too frequently, and over long periods of time, damage the body. You just need to be reminded again.

METHOTREXATE

Methotrexate is a antimetabolite which can be given by tablets or by injections. It basically inhibits folic acid in the form of dihydrofolic acid reductase. It interferes with DNA synthesis, repair and cellular replication. Active malignant cells, bone marrow, fetal cells, buccal and intestinal mucosa cells, cells of the urinary bladder are more sensitive to methotrexate.

Its mechanism of action in rheumatoid cases is unknown. It can stop pain, swelling and stiffness in the RA case but it doesn't cause remission of the disease, and it can't stop the growing deformities or joint degenerations.

Methotrexate has the potential for serious toxicity, which can occur at any time during therapy without warning. NSAIDS do intensify and destabilize the effects of methotrexate, which has resulted in some deaths.

Methotrexate's package insert starts with a **thick bordered _WARNING_**. The warnings cover two full pages. It says methotrexate should be used only by physicians whose knowledge and experience includes the use of antimetabolite therapy. Because of the possibility of serious toxic reactions the patient should be informed by the physician of the risks involved and should be under constant supervision.

Most physicians gloss over the side effects and the lethal hazards of this drug, fearing the patient will refuse to take it. The doctor's problem is they don't know where else to turn. What do you do next when the current drugs aren't working anymore and the patient is getting worse. You, as a doctor, know that methotrexate will work. You hope the patient won't be the one that develops the severe side effects that you know are possible. It's a hard choice for a doctor who is being asked for help by an obviously suffering patient.

Deaths have been reported with the use of methotrexate in the treatment of malignancy, psoriasis, and rheumatoid arthritis. If psoriasis or rheumatoid arthritis are being treated, methotrexate should be restricted to patients with severe, recalcitrant, disabling disease which is not adequately responding to other forms of therapy. Consultations with other physicians should also be done before the medicines are taken.

Methotrexate can cause fetal abnormalities and fetal death.

Periodic liver biopsies should be considered. Liver and renal function tests are mandatory. Methotrexate is known to cause hepatotoxicity, fibrosis and cirrhosis. Liver damage can occur without symptoms or changes in laboratory tests. Liver enzyme elevations are frequently seen.

Methotrexate may produce marked bone marrow depression with resultant anemia, leukopenia and thrombocytopenia. Diarrhea and ulcerative stomatitis require the discontinuation of treatment, otherwise hemorrhagic enteritis and death from intestinal perforation may occur. Unexpectedly severe (sometimes fatal) marrow suppression and gastrointestinal toxicity have been reported with methotrexate, along with NSAIDS.

Permanent and semi-permanent neurological changes can occur such as behavioral changes and abnormal reflexes. Methotrexate can also cause malaise, fatigue, chills and fever, dizziness, and decreased resistance to infections.

It can cause gastrointestinal ulceration and bleeding, headaches, drowsiness, blurred vision, aphasia, hemiparesis, and convulsions.

Methotrexate can cause everything from gingivitis to vomiting blood, headaches, paresis, blurred vision, interstitial pneumonitis with deaths, rashes, boils, alopecia, spiderveins and acne.

And the list goes on—Methotrexate can cause severe kidney damage, menstrual dysfunctions, vaginal discharge, infertility, loss of libido, diabetes, osteoporosis and sudden death without cause. Not to mention cirrhosis, anemia, tinnitus.

. . . and they don't even know why methotrexate is so toxic.

Although the predominantly anti-inflammatory actions of methotrexate do control chronic polyarthritis, in most cases where it's used, methotrexate is unable to prevent the primarily immunological tissue necrosis. . . and may even promote its development.

There is a recent report, for example, of a 58-year-old woman with chronic polyarthritis who rapidly developed a large number of rheumatic nodules **while on methotrexate**. For the nodules (which are common to rheumatoid patients) to become suddenly worse means the drug was actually *causing the condition* it was supposed to be healing.

NSAIDs

Non-steroidal anti-inflammatory drugs are called NSAIDs. They exhibit anti-inflammatory, antipyretic and analgesic pharmacological properties. No one really can say how they work, the same as for methotrexate. It is believed they may inhibit prostaglandin synthesis.

Here is a place to remind you that no one knows how 60% to 70% of the current drugs work, and yet millions of them are prescribed daily. Two of the major uses are for rheumatoid and osteoarthritis.

I don't know how *CMO* works either, but I know it has virtually no side effects to worry about. That cannot be said about prescription drugs.

Elderly patients have to be careful of overdoses, and people with liver damage should be careful, as NSAIDs are degraded by the liver. Some of them increase bleeding time.

Liver function tests may become abnormal. Severe hepatic reactions, including jaundice and fatal hepatitis have been reported. Fluid retention and edema are common.

NSAIDs damage the gastrointestinal tract. High risk patients, such as the elderly, or those with previous ulcers, or those on cortisone should think twice before using.

One of the greatest dangers is gastrointestinal ulceration,

bleeding and perforation of the gut. It can occur anytime and without warning in patients using NSAIDS, non-steroidal anti-inflammatory drugs. Ulcers as a result of these treatments are not rare. The doctor is supposed to warn you of these hazards but my experience is that they usually don't.

There is a long list of possible side effects. Virtually any gastrointestinal problem can occur: diarrhea, dyspepsia, constipation, gas, nausea, gastritis and vomiting. Jaundice, gastroenteritis, increased hunger, gallstones, glossitis, pancreatitis, and rectal bleeding.

Central nervous system symptoms might include dizziness, headaches, fatigue, insomnia, nervousness, tinnitis, agitation, anxiety, confusion, depression, malaise, paresthesia, tremor, vertigo and nightmares.

Dermatological symptoms include: photosensitivity, acne, alopecia, pruritus, rash,

One can have angioneurotic edema, anaphylaxis, vasculitis and weight gain. Hypoglycemia, low potassium, anemia, fever, chills and taste disorder.

Respiratory symptoms include dyspnea, pneumonitis, asthma and cough.

Urinary symptoms includes albumin in the urine, vaginal bleeding, burning and pain on urination, blood in the urine and renal stones. And impotency.

Long-term administration runs the risk of renal papillary necrosis and other abnormal renal pathology. There is also the possibility that they can reduce the blood flow through the kidneys.

An unusual component of a lipid was found in heart tissue after treatment with a NSAID. Here is a good example of what I am saying. Rheumatoid arthritics have plenty to worry about if they are planning on taking anti-rheumatic drugs for any period of time: the danger is "Silent Heart Disease". An underlying disease like this can occur even in the absence of symptoms.

The European Heart Journal reported in February 1995 that arthritics develop posterior pericardial effusion, aortic root alterations and thickening of the valves of the heart, all of which take place without the patient knowing it. They have named this condition the "Silent Rheumatoid heart."

GOLD

Reactions to gold injections: Nitritoid and vasomotor reactions have been encountered with all therapeutic gold compounds. Most of the time these symptoms have been mild, but not always. Some patients have had heart attacks, while others have had strokes.

No reasonable person could read the literature on these drugs and still insist they are the ultimate answer for chronic diseases.

Now you can see why it is necessary that *CMO* and similar agents reach the public's attention.

This information has to come down like a hammerhead in order to thwack the public and get its attention.

26

QUESTIONS
AND ANSWERS

WHO CAN TAKE THIS PRODUCT?

Just about everyone can take this product. You've read the side effects and you know the risks are small.

CAN YOU TAKE *CMO* IF YOU HAVE NO SYMPTOMS OF A DISEASE?

I think you can. It could be especially helpful as a prevention for sports injuries. It could be helpful if you are a weekend warrior, jogger or bicycler. It's good insurance against an injury.

HOW STABLE IS FISH OIL?

Since it is an oil, by inference it might become rancid and oxidize when exposed to air, light or heat. An experiment was done to determine if this was true and then published in Nutrition and Cancer, 1992. Rat chow powdered diet was analyzed for fatty acid oxidation. Four samples were taken during a 45-day period. There was no appreciable difference in the oil from the 4th day to the 45th day.

IS THERE A BETTER TREATMENT PROTOCOL?

You've undoubtedly ask yourself this question during the course of reading this book. How do the doctors know which dosage schedules work best for *CMO*? How do they know that two weeks of treatment, is the best approach to each health problem? The answer is they don't. The present treatment plan was simply an arbitrary decision based on some experiences with people. No one knows for sure whether better protocols are possible. The only thing we know for sure is that the desired response is never enough without at least two weeks of stimulation. A more efficient approach may certainly be possible.

At the present time I am placing my new patients on two capsules, three times a day.

SHOULD WE LIMIT OUR DIET WHILE ON *CMO*?

Should we use a diet along with *CMO* or do we even need one? In some cases I'm sure that would be the right thing to do.

Should we repeat the series from time to time? In many cases that would seem appropriate. Only time and experience will answer these questions. With a larger number of doctors using this product, no doubt the protocol will be improved.

WILL CO-NUTRIENTS BE HELPFUL?

No one knows if the addition of other nutrients would improve the potency of *CMO*. Obviously I think it should: this has been the case with the essential fatty acids. Fish oil has enhanced the effectiveness of a number of drugs. As far as I know it has never undermined a drug's effectiveness.

The same thing is true when fish oil is combined with other nutrients, such as coenzyme Q 10. Coenzyme Q 10 and fish oil are powerful agents against a number of diseases. Why shouldn't they be used together?

I have already combined **CMO** with other non-drug treatments and found the combination to be superior to the use of either agent separately. I think complementary agents greatly increase the possibilities for success.

IF THE TWO WEEK TREATMENT WERE REPEATED, WOULD IT HELP?

There are a few hints as to the need for this adjustment. When patients repeat the series they often pick up another 10% to 20% improvement in symptoms. I have already tried this with good success.

You may ask, why bother? If everybody is cured what else is there to do. Think back. I said many of the patients had 70% improvements. If I had a serious disease and I had a 70% improvement, I'd want to do more about my problem if more could be done. I would be happy to repeat the protocol to finally be free of the whole mess. I am quite certain that enhancing **CMO**'s effect is possible.

Let me repeat something I said earlier in the book, when I was discussing the response of rats to **CETYL MYRISTOLEATE** injections. In one case, Diehl injected **CETYL MYRISTOLEATE** into the back of a susceptible rat before administering the arthritis causing toxin. In spite of the injection of **CETYL MYRISTOLEATE** several rats developed arthritis in one of their feet. Diehl thought that if **CETYL MYRISTOLEATE** had been injected in the foot the arthritis would probably not developed where it did. He thought **CETYL MYRISTOLEATE** had simply not dispersed itself enough to reach all areas of the body.

Here's why. . . **CETYL MYRISTOLEATE** was injected in mineral oil, and we know that both oils should have been evenly throughout the body. Both oils were especially strong in the liver as expected, but, in some cases where the arthritis developed in susceptible rats it was found that **CETYL MYRISTOLEATE** had not made it's way to the affected foot but the mineral oil had. It was suspected then that the location of the injection made a difference in whether arthritis would develop or not.

This observation makes one wonder if **CETYL MYRISTOLEATE** may not always be dispersed through the body uniformly in all patients. And this may be the reason there is some variability in success. Some patients reach 100% improvement while others reach only 70%. That's a difference of 30%, or one-third; that's a big enough difference to be concerned about.

WOULD VITAMIN E HELP *CMO*?

Vitamin E is the major fat-soluble, chain-breaking antioxidant in biological membranes and protects membrane EFAs from lipid peroxidation. The requirements for vitamin E rise as the use of EFAs rises. Adequate levels of vitamin E are needed for normal function of the immune cells.

DOES FISH OIL HAVE SIDE EFFECTS?

There is one drawback to taking large amounts of fish oil, which seems to be even worse in older people. Too much fish oil can actually depress the immune system. That's alright and just what you want when you have an overactive immune system contributing to a chronic disease. It's not so great if you are the kind that catches everything.

Another thing is that too much fish oil can cause a vitamin E deficiency. That's because fish oil (n-3) requires vitamin E to make its effect. You can use up a lot of E in a short time if you are pushing the fish oil limits.

The bottom line is that if you are going to increase your fish oil, then increase your vitamin E also. 400-800 units of E should be enough.

SHOULD CHILDREN TAKE *CMO*?

I don't think it would hurt, it may do them enormous good, but I can not advise it at this time.

DOES IT MAKE ANY DIFFERENCE WHAT TIME OF THE DAY I TAKE *CMO*?

No, but it should be on an empty stomach. It's probably not a good idea to take it too late in the day as many say it's a real stimulant.

IF I'M TAKING HEART MEDICINES IS IT ALRIGHT TO TAKE *CMO*?

I would give it to any of my patients without worry, I've done it many times: ask your doctor first, of course. I did not say it was safe to take <u>if you have a heart disease that you are not being treated for</u>.

I HAVE AN IRREGULAR HEART BEAT, IS *CMO* SAFE IN THIS CASE?

Don't take *CMO* unless your doctor says you can.

IS *CMO* SAFE DURING PREGNANCY?

Don't take *CMO* during pregnancy unless your doctor agrees you can.

There is one recent case of a patient becoming pregnant one week after taking *CMO* for another problem. She had been unable to conceive for 10 years durning which time she had numerous medical treatments.

CAN *CMO* BE TAKEN IF I HAVE SEVERE ALLERGIES?

I advise against it, but you might seek out an experienced physician and discuss it with him.

I HAVE A SEVERE HORMONE DISTURBANCE, IS *CMO* SAFE?

CMO is probably safe and may even help, but you should be under a doctors supervision.

WILL INSURANCE PAY FOR *CMO*?

I doubt it. It is not a prescribable drug on any acceptable list. The sad thing is—if it were a drug they would pay, but since its a natural substance they won't.

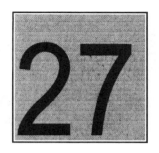

RESOURCES AND REVIEW

This Chapter will include a source for **CMO** and the other nutritional items mentioned in the book. I will also add a few tips.

CMO is not a prescription item, so it's not necessary to be under a physician's care to use it. However, I advise you to use **CMO** under the supervision of a knowledgeable physician. You will have a better chance for a satisfactory outcome if you do.

SOURCES FOR THE NUTRIENTS MENTIONED IN "BOOM—YOU'RE WELL"

CETYL MYRISTOLEATE (*CMO*)
KNOLLWOOD, INC. 800-249-7816

CETYL MYRISTOLEATE FOR LONG-TERM USE
(KNOLLWOOD - see above)

Super oxide dismutase (SOD)
    GERO VITA 800-694-8366

Prostata
    GERO VITA 800-694-8366

Sphingolin and Rheumatoid factor (collagen type two)
    Ecological Research 800-888-4585

Medium chain fatty acids
    Life Enhancement 800-543-3873

Kool and Fit
    Kool and Fit 800-852-5655

Guaifenesin
    Apothecure 800-969-6601

Vanadyl Sulfate
    Apothecure 800-969-6601

Injectable thymus
    Apothecure 800-969-6601

SIDE EFFECTS

I've treated many people with *CMO* and seldom seen side effects, and yet there have been a few, which I will now review.

CONSTIPATION

I have seen this in a handful of patients.
It always clears up the day after *CMO* is stopped.
Herbal laxatives overcome it.

LOOSE STOOLS

I Have only seen this once: however, it is not uncommon to have yellow or greenish stools. If your feces turns another color don't become alarmed, it's not harmful.

ABDOMINAL PAIN OR DISCOMFORT

This is rare, usually occurring in an individual with an ulcer or a past history of ulcer-like activity. You may have to discontinue the *CMO* entirely, or try it in smaller amounts. If you decide to try smaller amounts, use this formula. Equal parts of table sugar and Maalox, and some powder from a capsule of *CMO*.

ALLERGIES

Sometimes *CMO* makes allergies worse. The symptoms reverse once *CMO* is discontinued. If you have allergies, you must start on a much lower dose to test the waters. Oddly enough, some allergic people lose their allergies with *CMO*. This is a gray area at the moment.

ASTHMA

I strongly recommend you **do not use** *CMO* except under a doctors supervision. I have heard of some individuals benefiting from *CMO*, but I have personally seen people with asthma get seriously worse.

PROSPECTIVE

The way I see it, *CMO* is like a stage actor, taking the lead role in some diseases and a supporting role in others. *CMO* has a leading role in rheumatoid arthritis or prostate enlargement. It has a supporting role in autoimmune diseases. Sometimes it's more like the theater itself—not a part of the play but there to allow the play to happen. *CMO* may act this way in hypertension, diabetes and aging.

CMO has more of a lasting effect than the EFAs, but its reserve can be exhausted too. EFAs, like all nutrients, are being consumed daily and require constant replacement. Nutritionists believe that a good healthy diet is enough, and that supplements are not necessary. The presence of a chronic disease changes the equation though, because the body's defenses consume more EFAs than a normal diet can provide.

Nutritional deficiencies found in the aged make it clear that food alone is enough to cover the shortages. Evidence grows that EFA replacement is less efficient as one ages. Elderly individuals who appear perfectly normal are often found to be deficient in EFAs. And since EFAs are necessary defenders of the antioxidant system, it's easy to see how other systems are off-balanced as well.

EFAs have a very short life in the body, perhaps even as little as a day or two. *CMO*, on the other hand, seems to have a longer life in the body. Not having been the subject of such intense study as EFAs have been, it's pure speculation and impossible to make firm statements about *CMO*. I have only my personal observations to go by, plus the input from others who are relaying their observations to me.

It appears to me that *CMO* is an undiscovered essential nutrient that is important for the body's defense. Unless you eat beaver tails or sperm whales I don't know how you would get enough of it in you diet, although **CETYL MYRISTOLEATE** is supposed to be in grains and vegetables (in minute quantities). Disease, aging and stress exhaust *CMO* exactly like they exhaust the EFAs.

Since *CMO* is a nutrient of importance in the body, I think it should be used by everybody after age 55. I think it is depleted as we grow older allowing us to become susceptible to degenerative diseases. Undoubtedly there are important interrelated cofactors to be discovered: time and experience will bring them to light.

I think, because **CMO** is as natural a nutrient as vitamin C, the public should have free access to it. Research funds should be allocated immediately for the investigation of benefits derived from **CMO**. If **CMO** is seized by an *alphabet bureaucrat,* as may happen once they realize that something new is out there they don't control, then they have pounded another nail in the coffin of freedom. What we need for better health, if that happens, is full and complete protection against an oppressive government. We don't need protection against vitamins, we need protection against **control freaks**.

I THINK **CMO** IS THE FIRST MAJOR NUTRITIONAL DISCOVERY OF THE CENTURY. Who knows what the limits are to its power?

FORECAST

I warn you the ideas presented here will meet with enormous opposition from the established fields of science. They will not be pleased they have been bypassed. They would love to have this product and slowly percolate it down through their ranks over a number of years. 20 years from now they would gradually release this wonder nutrient to the public through the medical networks with their endless rituals.

Unfortunately those who are desperate for it **_now_** will probably be dead, or so old and crippled they no longer care what happens to them. Paradoxically, if the product is free for the public's use, now and into the future, most of those who need it will still be around and in good shape.

ABOUT THE AUTHOR

Douglas Hunt M.D., completed his undergraduate work at U.C.L.A. and received his medical degree from the University of California at Irvine. Since 1965 he has dedicated his time to the study and use of alternative care approaches to health. He is author of NO MORE CRAVINGS, which was published by Warner Books. NO MORE CRAVINGS was sold through the Rodale Book Club. In addition, Dr. Hunt is author of NO MORE FEARS, which was also published by Warner Books.

Dr. Hunt lectures to numerous business and professional groups and is a well-known speaker on the subjects of weight control, aging and alternative care medicine. He gives weekly lectures on nutrition, focusing on the importance of daily preventive care to insure a physically healthy future. Dr. Hunt practices in Burbank, California, and his work includes attending to the health needs of many active studio executives and entertainers who rely on physical stamina for success.

Dr. Hunt is also a well-known media personality. For a while he hosted a radio program for KIEV in Los Angeles called "Alive in L.A." Now he can now be heard weekly on the Jim Leche radio talk show which airs on KBET in Los Angeles. Dr. Hunt is currently negotiating for a new show called "Alternative Care Solutions" on a radio station KKLA which reaches most of Southern California.

After the publication of NO MORE CRAVINGS, producers from the popular morning talk show "A.M. L.A." asked Dr. Hunt to treat three of their staff members who were overweight and bring them on periodically to weigh and measure the results. After eight weeks Dr. Hunt appeared on the final program with his three thin "graduates."

Subsequently, after the publication of NO MORE FEARS, "A.M. L.A." asked Dr. Hunt to treat two patients with phobias, then bring them on live television to be interviewed. He successfully treated one patient for fear of heights and another for free-floating anxiety, and their appearance together on "A.M. L.A." made an exciting and successful program.

Throughout his career, Dr. Hunt has been faithful to his strong belief in exploring alternatives to traditional drug therapy. *CMO* has proven to be another success story for Dr. Hunt. It's a safe and superior replacement for drugs.

Dr. Hunt is one of the few doctors in the country to start the *CMO* trend. This early start allowed him to have more clinical experience with *CMO* than most doctors, and, in addition, he is in direct contact with all of the major clinics who use it.

Why did Dr. Hunt write this book? Every time he told one patient about some benefit received by a fellow patient using *CMO,* they would say, "Oh, I know someone who could use that." I think everybody knows someone (or more than one) who has been struggling with a chronic disease and losing the fight; nothing speaks louder than a testimonial, and there are plenty of those in this book.

REFERENCES

Olivieri O; Stanzial A.M.; Girelli D; Trevisan M.T.; Guarini P; Terzi M; Caffi S; Fontana F; Casaril M; Ferrari S. (1995). Selenium status, fatty acids, vitamins A and E, and aging. American Journal of Clinical Nutrition, 61(5):1174.

Drainev A.G.; Ferrington D.A.; Williams T.D.; Squier T.C.; Bigelow D.J. (1995). Adaptive changes in lipid composition of skeletal sarcoplasmic reticulum membranes associated with ageing. Biochimica et Biophysica Acta, 1235(2):406-18.

Driessens F.C.M. (1994). Theory of aging in humans and hypotheses about its possible delay. Medical Hypotheses, 43, 187-92.

Smith R.S. (1992). The cytokine theory of headache. Medical Hypotheses, 39(2):168-74.

Stevens R.J.; Hughes R.A. (1995). The aetiopathogenesis of giant cell arteritis. British Journal of Rheumatology, 34:960-65.

Williams L.L.; Kiecolt-Glaser J.K.; Horrocks L.A.; Hillhouse J.T.; Glaser R. (1992). Quantitative association between altered plasma esterified omega-6 fatty acid proportions and psychological stress. Prostaglandins Leukotrienes and Essential Fatty acids, 47(2):165-70.

Holden R.J.; Mooney P.A. (1994). Schizophrenia is a diabetic brain state: an elucidation of impaired neurometabolism. Medical Hypotheses, 43(6):420-35.

Bourre J.M.; Bonneil M.; Chaudiere J.; Clement M.; Dumont O.; Durand G.; Lafont H.; Nalbone G.; Pascal G.; Piciotti M. (1992). Structural and functional importance of dietary polyunsaturated fatty acids in the nervous system. Advances in Experimental Medicine and Biology, 318:211-29.

Yao J.K.; van Kammen D.P.; Gurklis J. (1994). Red blood cell membrane dynamics in schizophrenia. Correlation of fatty acid abnormalities with clinical measures. Schizophrenia Research, 13(3):227-32.

Hibbeln J.R.; Salem N. (1995). Dietary polyunsaturated fatty acids and depression: when cholesterol does not satisfy. American Journal of Clinical Nutrition, 62(1):1-9.

Bierenbaum M.L.; Chen Y.; Lei H.; Watkins T. (1992). Relationship between dietary fatty acid, selenium, and degenerative cardiomyopathy. Medical Hypotheses, 39(1): 58-62.

Chidambaram N.; Baradarajan A. (1995). Effects of selenium on lipids and some lipid metabolising enzymes in DMBA induced mammary tumor rats. Cancer Biochemestry Biophysics, 15(1):41-7.

Crespo A.M.; Reis M.A.; Lanca M.J. (1995). Effect of selenium supplementation on polyunsaturated fatty acids in rats. Biological Trace Element Research, 47(1-3):335-41.

Olivieri O.; Stanzial A.M.; Girelli D.; Trevisan M.T.; Guarini P.; Terzi M.; Caffi S.; Fontana F.; Casaril M.; Ferrari S., et al. (1994). Selenium status, fatty acids, vitamins A and E, and aging: the Nove Study. American Journal of Clinical Nutrition, 60(4):510-7.

Huang K.; Lauridsen E.; Clausen J. (1994). The uptake of Na-selenite in rat brain. Localization of new glutathione peroxidases in the rat brain. Biological Trace Element Research, 46(1-2):91-102.

Sakurai H.; Fumii K.; Watanobe H.; Tamura H. (1995). Orally active and long-term acting insulin-mimetic vanadyl complex. Biochemical and Biophysical Research, 214(3):1095-101.

Nakai M.; Watanabe H.; Fujiwara C.; Kakegawa H.; Satoh T.; Takada J.; Matsushita R.; Sakurai H. (1995). Mechanism on insulin-like action of vanadyl sulfate: studies on interaction between rat adipocytes and vanadium compounds. Biological and Pharmaceutical Bulletin, 18(5):719-25.

Becker D.J.; Ongemba L.N.; Henquin J.C. (1994). Comparison of the effects of various vanadium salts on glucoles homeostasis in streptozotocin-diabetic rats. European Journal of Pharmacology, 260(2-3):169-75.

Ozcelikay A.T.; Pekiner C.; Ari N.; Ozturk Y.; Ozuari A.; Altan V.M. (1994). The effect of vanadyl treatment on vascular responsiveness of streptozotocin-diabetic rats. Diabetologia, 37(6):572-8.

Dai S.; Thompson K.H.; McNeill J.H. (1994). One-year treatment of streptozotocin-induced diabetic rats with vanadyl sulphate. Pharmacology and Toxicology, 74(2):101-9.

Bhanot S.; McNeill J.H. (1994). Vanadyl sulfate lowers plasma insulin and blood pressure in spontaneously hypertensive rats. Hypertension, 24(5):625-32.

McCarty M.F. (1994). Insulin resistance - not hyperinsulinemia - is pathogenic in essential hypertension. Medical Hypotheses, 42:226-36.

Jacob C.; Belleville T. (1992). L-carnatine: metabolism, functions and value in pathology. Pathologie Biologie, 40(9):910-9.

Pierrefiche G.; Reynier M.; Laborit H. (1993). Carnitine action on neuromuscular disturbances in the fasting rat: potentiation by L-lysine. Pharmacology, 46(1):33-42.

Igisu H.; Matsuoka M.; Iryo Y. (1995). Protection of the brain by carnitine. Sangyo Eiseigaku Zasshi, 37(2):75-82.

Cotter M.A.; Cameron N.E.; Keegan A.; Dines K.C. (1995). Effects of acetyl- and proprionyl-L-carnatine on peripheral nerve function and vascular supply in experimental diabetes. Metabolism: Clinical and Experimental, 44(9):1209-14.

Maturo J., Dulakowski E.C. Insulin-like activity of Taurine. Taurine: Biological Actiona and Clinical Perspectives, eds. Oja S.S., Ahtee L., Kontro P., Paasonen M.K. Allan R. Lis, Inc. N.Y.

Yan C.C.; Bravo E.; Cantafora A. (1993). Effect of taurine levels on liver lipid metabolism: an in vivo study in the rat. Proceedings of the Society for Experimental Biology and Medicine, 202(1):88-96.

Gandhi V.M.; Cherian K.M.; Mulky M.J. (1992). Hypolipidemic action of taurine in rats. Indian Journal of Experimental Biology, 30(5):413-7.

Wang Q.; Hyde D.M.; Giri S.N. (1992). Abatement of Bleomycin-induced inc. In vascular permieability, inflammatory cell infiltration, and fibrotic lesions in hamster lungs by combined treatment with taurine and niacin. Laboratory Investigation, 67(2):234-42.

Stevens M.J.; Lattimer S.A.; Kamijo M.; Van Huysen C.; Sima A.A.; Greene D.A. (1993). Osmotically-induced nerve taurine depletion and the compatible osmolytic hypothesis in experimental diabetic neuropathy in the rat. Diabetologia, 36(7):608-14.

Azuma J.; Sawamura A.; Awata N. (1992). Usefulnesss of taurine in chronic congestive heart failure and it's prospective application. Japanese Circulation Journal, 56(1):95-9.

Fujita T.; Sato Y. (1987). Hypotensive effect of taurine. Possible involvement of the sympathetic nervous system and endogenous opiates. Journal of Clinical Investigation, 82(3):993-7.

Fujita T.; Ando K.; Noda H.; Ito Y.; Sato Y. (1987). Effects of increased adrenomedullary activity and taurine in young patients with borderline hypertension. Circulation, 75(3):525-32.

Fujita T.; Sato Y.; Ando K. (1987). Role of sympathetic nervous system in hypotensive action of taurine in DOCA-salt rats. Hypertension, 9(1):81-7.

Raffaele De. (1994). Effects of Fatty Acids and Lipids in Health and Disease. Basel, Karger, vol 76, 130-132.

DeMarco D.M.; Santoli D.; Zurier R.B. (1994). Effects of fatty acids on proliferation and activation of humanm synovial compartment lymphocytes. Journal of Leukocyte Biology, 56(5):612-5.

Calder P.C.; Bevan S.J.; Newsholme E.A. (1992). The inhibition of T-lymphocyte proliferation by fatty acids is via an eicosanoid-independent mechanism. Immunology, 75(1):108-15.

Purasiri P.; Ashby J.; Heys S.D.; Eremin O. (1994). Effect of essential fatty acids on circulating T cell subsets in patients with colorectal cancer. Cancer Immunology, Immunotherapy, 39(4): 217-22.

Soyland E.; Nenseter M.S.; Braathen L.; Drevon C.A. (1993). Very long chain n-3 and n-6 polyunsaturated fatty acids inhibit proliferation of human T-lymphocytes in vitro. European Journal of Clinical Investigation, 23(2):112-21.

Zurier R.B. (1993). Fatty acids, inflammation and immune responses. Prostaglandins Leukotrienes and Essential Fatty Acids, V 48:57-62.

Moosbrugger I.; Bischoff P.; Beck J.P.; Luu B.; Borg J. (1992). Studies on the immunological effects of Fatty alcohols. International Journal of Immunopharmacology, V14, No2. pp 293-302.

Cronstein B.N.; Naime D.; Firestein G. (1995). The antiinflammatory effects of adenosine kinase inhibitor are mediated by adenosine. Arthritis and Rheumatism, 38(8):1040-5.

Cronstein B.N. (1994). Adenosine, an endogenous anti-inflammatory agent. Journal of Applied Physiology, 76(1):5-13.

Grimble R.F. (1994). Nutritional antioxidants and the modulation of inflammation: theory and practice. New Horizons, 2(2):175-85.

Kamp F.; Zakim D.; Zhang F.; Noy N.; Hamilton J.A. (1995). Fatty acid flip-flop in phospholipid bilayers is extremely fast. Biochemistry, 34(37):11928-37.

Trentham D.E.; Dynesius-Trentham R.A.; orav E.J.; Combitchi D.; Lorenzo C.; Sewell K.L.; Hafler D.A.; Weiner H.L. (1993). Effects of Oral administration of type 2 collagen on rheumatoid arthritis. Science, V 261:1727-30.

Endres S.; Sinha B. (1994). The Effects of Fatty Acids and Lipids in Health and Disease. Basel, Karger, vol 76, pp 89-94.

Tvrzick E.; Cvrckova E.; Maca B.; Jiraskova M. (1995). The effect of ibuprofen on the composition of tissue lipids in an experiment. Casopis Lekaru Ceskych, 134(14):450-5.

Hill C.; Pile K.; Henderson D.; Kirkham B. (1995). Neurological side effects in two patients receiving gold injections for rheumatoid arthritis. British Journal of Rheumatology, 34:989-990.

ADDITIONAL INFORMATION

Dr. Hunt now offers personal consultations by telephone on any nutritional subject. **818-566-9889**

The charge is $3.00 per minute (subject to change) billed to your Master Card, Visa or AMEX. You may speak any length of time.

Dr. Hunt offers a newsletter "Boom, You're Well" which covers the entire nutritional field including Cetyl Myristoleate and aging.

Also available are books, special reports and pamphlets.

Dr. Hunt is available for press and media interviews and to speak to some special interest groups.